Dear Reader,

If I were to ask a hundred people why they picked up this book, I'd probably hear a hundred different reasons. But there is a common thread that can be found in one word—searching. Searching. Searching for what? For peace, for renewal, for joy, for love . . . you know best what it is you are searching for.

What *I* know is that there is something in the words "Reconnecting to the Magic of Life" that has drawn your attention. In truth, the entire content of this book is in the quiet, personal spaces between those words. *Reconnecting . . . to the Magic . . . of Life.*

I will show you ways to rediscover these spaces, to find them, and to reclaim them. I will tell you some stories. In these stories there are parts of you, of me, of those who came before, of those who have not yet arrived. And it is in the resonance that profound learning happens, that reconnection begins to take root.

I will also show you some essential stretching exercises. These exercises are designed not to help you touch your toes, but to encourage you to touch the sky. They work those muscles that are so often neglected, those that allow us to see beyond the frustrations of daily life. The stories reveal; the exercises allow you to internalize revelation.

In the end, *Reconnecting to the Magic of Life* is a guide to new beginnings. As you close the book, you will find that your heart and mind have become more open—that they can open again and again, no matter what the world slings at you, ever hopeful, ever more.

Joyce Mills

Also by Joyce C. Mills

Mills, Joyce C. & Crowley, Richard J. (1986). *Therapeutic Metaphors for Children and the Child Within.* New York: Brunner/Mazel, Publishers, a member of the Taylor & Francis Group.

Mills, Joyce C. (1992). *Little Tree: A Story for Children with Serious Medical Problems.* Washington, DC: Magination Press.

Mills, Joyce C. (1993). *Gentle Willow: A Story for Children About Dying.* Washington, DC: Magination Press.

Mills, Joyce C. & Crowley, Richard J. (1988). *Sammy the Elephant and Mr. Camel.* Washington, DC: Magination Press.

Mills, Joyce C. (1989). *Stories of the Dreamwalkers* (Limited Edition). Distributed by author. Kekaha, HI.

Crowley, Richard J. & Mills, Joyce C. (1989). *Cartoon Magic: How to Help Children Discover Their Rainbows Within.* Washington, DC: Magination Press.

Reconnecting

to the

Magic

of *Life*

Joyce C. Mills, Ph.D.

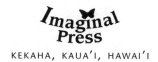

Imaginal
Press

KEKAHA, KAUA'I, HAWAI'I

Published by
Imaginal Press
PO Box 1109
Kekaha, Kaua'i, HI 96752

Manufactured in the United States of America.

10 9 8 7 6 5 4 3 2 1

Dedication

To the loving memory of my beautiful mother, Rose,
who gave me the precious gift of life.
To the wisdom teachings of my Bubbie Fannie.
To the laughter of the children . . .
and
To the stories already told and to the stories yet to be.

Acknowledgments

It is with the fullness of love and gratitude in my heart that I thank each of these special relatives, friends, and clients whose dedicated love, friendship, trust, and support provided me with the foundation upon which all of my life's blessings and teachings rest.

First, to my loving husband, Eddie, whom I met one December day back in 1959 in Philadelphia while dancing on American Bandstand. To the dances we have danced and to the dances yet to come. May we always hear the music of the heart.

To my precious sons, Todd and Casey, whose patience, understanding, and love fill the canvas of my life with beauty, challenge, and meaning. To Lynette and Tyler, who bring added joy and sunshine to Casey's life and to the life of our family.

To my sister, Rosalie, who showed me unconditional love when I most needed it. To my Aunt Bebe and my cousin Helene, who are always there in ways of the heart.

To Bernie Mazel, an angel in my life. His generosity of friendship and continued faith in this book shall forever hold a sacred place within my heart.

To Natalie Gilman, whose astute editorial guidance, patience, honesty, and friendship brought this book to fruition. To Suzi Tucker, whose artistic eye and gifted knowledge of production transformed my visualization of this book into a reality.

To my brother in spirit, Dr. Carl Hammerschlag, a true healer . . . a wisdom teacher in my life who openly shares his heartsongs . . . always reminding me to "look again," and "above all not to fear."

To Mona Polacca, CharlesEtta Sutton, Elaine Hammerschlag, Andrea Luna, and my beautiful Turtle Island sisters, who continually touch my life with wisdom, blessings, healing, and love.

Acknowledgments

To my treasured "Ya-Ya Sisters," Gail Sebern, Penee Hochman, and Rita Silverman . . . to the births, the deaths, and the beauty we have shared along the way.

To Richard Crowley, a soulmate, friend, and spiritual brother, who showed me how to reconnect with my own playful self and color outside the lines.

To Barbara Harris, Charles Weingarten, Thomas Hamlin, Brian Sebern, Herb Silverman, Jeff Hochman, Bernie and Harriet Bernard, Mike Sapp, Linda Berdeski, Cristina Whitehawk, Barbara Sinclair, Barbara Gordon, Lynn Langford, Philippe Eichhorn, and Irma Bollinger, and to the many hidden angels of friendship who so generously shared their ideas, provided support, and touched my life in quiet ways so that this book could be born.

To those relatives of spirit who continue to bless my life with their sacred tribal teachings of vision and prayer: Jerry and Mazie Nelson, Agnes and Yazzie Todechine, Jennifer Curtis-Skeets, Thomas and Violet Curtis, Nelson Fernandez, Terry Tafoya, George Eagle Man, Art McConville, Arvol Looking Horse, and Barbara, Arlana, and Arlo Omaha.

To Kalani Flores, Malia and David Fu, Grandpa Charlie Fu, Aunty Martha Kruse, Ray and Rose Peters, Tommy and Una Mae Kuhlmann, Lani Kaeo Apo, Wahinekula LaCro, and Abraham Martin, whose stories and friendship have helped to bring a rainbow into my life in the midst of a great storm.

To Sister Katherine Knoll, Jeraldene Lovell, John MacFarland, Ken Rutherford, Arun and Sunanda Gandhi, Jill Hagen, Diana Linden, Naomi Steinberg, Tami Sperle, Buffy Kane, Germaine Cook, Buddy Zukow, Aimee and Sophia McCullough, the children and staff at the Christie School, and the many special friends, children, families, and students whose stories have been woven into the fabric of this book.

To Jack Canfield, Nancy Napier, Dr. Bernie Siegel, and Sam Horn, whose kind generosity with their time, guidance, friendship, and support is appreciated deeply.

Acknowledgments

To Stephen Gilligan, Ernest Rossi, Jeffrey Zeig, Mark Tracten, Mark Barnes, Violet Oaklander, Dan Mahler, and the many professional colleagues, mentors, workshop sponsors, and conference organizers— both nationally and internationally—who have supported my teachings and learnings through the years.

To Georgia Ann Hughes, an insightful literary agent, whose support and keen editorial abilities helped this book develop its wings.

To K. C. Cowen, whose extraordinary patience and teaching expertise encouraged me to open my "Windows," allowing me to journey into the computer age. And to Charlie Bohn at Southpaw Builders, who helped me expand my tiny writing space without moving a beam.

I also owe a dept of gratitude to twenty-three publishers whose rejections only solidified my determination to continue writing and publish this book.

To the enduring memory of Anne Emery Kyllo, Gershon Tucker III, Darrell Apo, Alexis Anton Keilback, Uncle Arthur Kalani Kruse, Lokelani Martha Yoshimi Kruse, Susana Shino, Harrington Luna, Martin High Bear, Mahatma Gandhi, and the precious souls who may not have been mentioned by name who have gone on to the Spirit World.

And to the memory of Milton H. Erickson, whose teachings provide a pathway into the gardens of healing potentials within us all.

To each of you named, and to the many unnamed, I say "Thank you" with my heart.

To All My Relations
With Aloha

Contents

Contents

A Note from the Author:

In respect, and at the request of my Native American relatives, I have chosen to adjust and, in some cases, leave out specific details of the ceremonies mentioned in this book in order to protect and honor their sacredness.

I have also changed names in specific instances to protect those who have so generously shared their stories with me.

Foreword

Reconnecting to the Magic of Life is a poignant, funny, sometimes painful journey shared with us by an author who risks reaching deep down inside herself to tell a story—a story that she hopes will inspire us to tell our own.

Dr. Joyce Mills is an Ericksonian hypnotherapist and the author of a wonderful book about how to create therapeutic metaphors for children. We first met at a workshop I conducted at a professional conference that focused on integrating Ericksonian teachings and Native American philosophies of healing. At the close of the workshop, Joyce continued to ask how she could learn more about the philosophy of Native Americans and their transmission of wisdom through the oral tradition.

I do not generally encourage people to come to Indian country or to participate in Native ceremonies. Many Native Americans feel that their spiritual life is the only thing that still remains their own. The oral tradition requires time spent sitting around fires, singing songs, and appreciating the power of ceremony.

I try to dissuade people from undertaking this journey, but Joyce would not be denied. I invited her to a Turtle Island Project retreat. The project, a nonprofit foundation cofounded by Native and non-Native healers, pioneered the idea of using ritual and ceremony in healing as a practical application of the new science of psychoneuroimmunology, or mind/body/spirit medicine.

Joyce became intimately involved with the Turtle Island Project. Over the last decade, she has established close relationships and participated in sacred ceremonies with many Native American relatives.

Joyce understands the power of suggestion and the importance of healing stories.

In this book, Joyce brings her great diversity of learning together. You will find a range of resources, *steppingstones* as Joyce calls them, that will help you acknowledge where you may be feeling stuck in your life and then find ways out; you'll find how to confront fear and emerge with faith. By accepting our behaviors, thoughts, and feelings, even embracing them, we begin to create the possibility for new endings in our personal stories. Joyce shows us how to unearth our own resources by providing stories and experiences that can inspire vision and the ability to soar in our ever-changing world.

Reconnecting to the Magic of Life will help you share your own stories. Tell them around dinner tables and campfires—tell personal stories, tribal stories, biblical stories. In the telling, there is healing. Here is a book that can help you continue your journey with greater joy and hope.

Carl A. Hammerschlag, M.D.
Cofounder of the Turtle Island Project
1998 recipient of the National Caring Award
Author of *The Dancing Healers*, *The Theft of the Spirit*, and *Healing Ceremonies*.

Reconnecting
to the
Magic
of *Life*

. . . And That Reminds Me of a Story

"In the dust where we have buried the silent races . . . we have buried so much of the delicate magic of life."

—D. H Lawrence[1]

How did a Jewish kid born in the Bronx wind up sitting in a tipi in Arizona chanting Hebrew songs, preparing chicken soup and matzoh balls for my adopted Navajo relatives, and moving to Kaua'i after twenty-seven years of living in Los Angeles only to be "welcomed" by the most devastating storm to hit the Hawaiian Islands? Phew! As I think about it, I think it is all part of a greater Mystery than I, as a simple human being, can explain. Perhaps it is this Mystery that is the connection to that "delicate magic of life," as D. H. Lawrence calls it. I believe that one of the most important missions we have in this upcoming twenty-first century is to help ourselves and to help those with whom we work and live to reconnect to the magic of life.

In recent years, with the advent of the "techno-computer-explosion," it seems that we have become a society where we value *point* and *click* more than *touch* and *feel*. We must remember that *magic* is not simply in the press of a button as much as it is in the smell of a rose, in the touch of a newborn's skin, or in the sound of a child's giggling laughter. It is the appearance of a tear, a rainbow, and the first tiny heartbeat felt within the womb of an expectant mother.

The challenge becomes: How do we reconnect to the magic of life when life doesn't feel like magic? When life contains trauma, stress, and pain? When life presents what appear to be personal storms in the form of insensitivities, inequities, and assaults to our very souls? For me, this reconnection happens through story. Stories are the medicine of the Soul, which act like natural herbs for healing and self-discovery. As Jungian analyst and storyteller Clarissa Pinkola Estes[2] tells us, "Stories set the inner life into motion, and this is particularly important where the inner life is frightened, wedged, or cornered."

As far back as my childhood, I have always used stories to communicate. My mother used to tell me that when I was a little girl I talked with everyone on the subway and I would tell them stories . . . and surprisingly they would give us a seat or they would simply talk with us. She also reminded me that I used to give everything away. One time when I was about eight years old I gave a medal I had won in a children's art show to a girlfriend whose mother had recently died. I thought that if I gave her the best thing that I had, it would help her feel better. My friend accepted the gift and we sat on the stoop hugging for a long time. When my mother asked me why I did that I said, "because she needed it." Just as my friend needed the medal, people need the stories. We need them to help bring smiles into our lives when our lives are filled with tears.

Over the years my experiences with Native American people have taught me how to see every season in life as a potential story . . . a medicine that contains enormous healing agents. This is a particularly wonderful way for me to learn, because I am not someone who remembers charts or graphs. I don't trust quick-fix cures. I find myself gravitating towards people who share wisdom from life lived, not simply knowledge gleaned from the latest how-to books. I truly don't believe that most of us are looking for someone to tell us *how* to live our lives. I believe as mythologist Joseph Campbell says, "I think what we're seeking is an experience of being alive, so that our life experiences on the purely physical plane will have resonances within our own innermost being and reality, so that we actually feel the rapture of being alive." Stories provide a pathway for experience.

Integrating the principles of Milton H. Erickson, a psychiatrist who was noted for his masterful use of storytelling and hypnosis, along with my personal experiences with Native American teachings, I have used stories as the seeds around which all of my therapeutic work grew and continues to grow. A client tells me his or her problem, and after a few moments, an image would come into my mind that opens a doorway through which a story emerges. After listening to the stories, my clients would begin to solve their problems or find a healing message that acts as a "medicine" for their emotional pains. Whether the problems are about having the courage to speak up for one's self, or issues around loss, abuse, or trauma, stories provide a medicine that allows my clients to discover what is important to them in their quest for well-being.

I believe that what most of us are looking for is the ability to contact our own inner wisdom to find the solutions to our problems. Where do we find this inner wisdom? Through stories. But where do we get stories? Some stories come from myths and legends. Some stories come from our everyday life experiences with family, nature, and self. Wherever stories come from, one thing is for sure . . . we remember them. Once told, they can never be lost. They are the legacies by which human beings can stay connected to life and find healing.

In modern terms, storytelling can also be viewed as the *Internet of the soul*, linking us with worlds past, present, future, and magical. While working on my first book, *Therapeutic Metaphors for Children and the Child Within*,[3] my interest in storytelling and metaphor naturally led me into the research of how other cultures use these ancient ways of communication. I became absorbed in the tales of the Eastern teachings, such as Taoism, Zen Buddhism, and Hinduism, as well as in the stories of Native American people, the Bushmen of Africa, and parables of Hassidism. Each story becomes like a kernel on a giant ear of corn growing in a vast cornfield called *life*.

One Hassidic story I remember was told to me by a colleague during a workshop I was teaching on using metaphors for healing with children. The story features the Baal Shem Tov, a rabbi and storyteller whose wise life-teachings and miraculous deeds remain legendary after thousands of years. I share it with you as I heard it told:

> *Once, a long time ago, the Baal Shem Tov was being criticized by many fellow Rabbis. They felt many of his ways dishonored the Sabbath by encouraging singing and freedom. In fact they wondered if he and his followers were madmen.*
>
> *The Baal Shem was then questioned by one of the scholars and asked, "Don't you think this kind of teaching is wrong . . . don't you think it is false?" The Baal Shem Tov replied with a story. He said:*
>
> *"Once there was a wonderful wedding in this town. The house where*

the wedding was taking place was filled with joy and happiness. The musicians played glorious music and all inside danced with great merriment. Outside a man walked by and looked through a window. But all he saw were people jumping about, whirling and leaping through the air. He walked away from the house muttering to himself that this must truly be a house of madmen. Just then, one of the men from inside the house opened the windows which had been closed all this time. The man turned once again toward the house, for now he was able to hear the joyous music being played from within."

This story, which has been told in many ways, imparts an encouraging message. The message I heard from the Baal Shem Tov is that one needs to open the windows of the soul if one is to hear the music of the heart. It is not always easy to hear the music of our heart when we are confronted with adversity, pain, or trauma. But as Native American elders tell us, "We hear when we are ready to listen."

The stories, rituals and ceremonies, life philosophies and teachings of the Native American and Hawaiian people have become infused with my own Jewish cultural teachings, and with a vision of healing I have come to learn, embrace, live, and respect. It is simply stated that within all of life there is also mystery. That to think with the mind and not feel with the heart is like a surgeon going into the operating room without equipment. That our greatest vision comes from seeing the magic that exists in all of life.

The stories in this book are gleaned from many sources: personal, professional, nature, culture, and myth. They are stories that I have lived and stories that have been shared with me throughout my years of life and work with others. Together with specific exercises sculpted into what I call "steppingstones," I offer them to you to be used as "spiritual vitamins" to help you confront the fears that may overshadow your lives and discover the faith that resides in the silent spaces of your heart . . . to help you to see life's scars as markers of where you have been, not where you are going . . . to help you discover and rediscover joy, healing, and the inspiration to soar . . . and above all, to help you connect and reconnect to the resounding magic that exists in your own lives—your heartsongs.

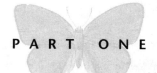

PART ONE

Renewal from the Roots Up

"Pay attention to the Wind, Listen to its voice."

—Hawaiian Proverb[1]

All of us live through hurricanes in one form or another, which force us into the process of change whether we are ready for it or not. Hurricanes can come in the form of life-challenging illness, the death of someone close, an unexpected accident, physical or sexual abuse, divorce, loss of livelihood—or, as experienced by millions around the world, in human-made or natural disasters.

These personal storms have the power to overturn the foundations of our beliefs and sever all sources of life's securities, as we have known them to be. Our dreams and passions can get lost in the turmoil of fear and trauma. If we let fear control our decisions and yearnings during these times of challenge, we can become disconnected from the magic that gives meaning and substance to living. By allowing fear a free reign, it will cast a shadow over every emerging idea and leave us emotionally paralyzed.

Fear has great importance, however. It can turn our attention towards something significant that is happening in our lives. Like the sirens that blast a warning signal before a hurricane, fear sends chemical signals throughout our bodies alerting us to possible impending dangers. However, fear is the messenger, *but not the message. The message is* faith. *And just what is faith? For me faith is believing . . . it is* being in life. *And* being in life *is the ability to take risks, confront our fears, and emerge with faith through it all.*

CHAPTER ONE

Fear Is the Messenger, Faith Is the Message

"Hope is a thing of feathers
That perches in the soul,
And sings the tune without the words,
And never stops at all. . . . "

— Emily Dickinson[2]

Have you ever fantasized about giving it all up to move to a tropical paradise where life is simpler and slower? Where suits and ties are rarely worn and dressing for power means a new pair of shorts and a matching flowered shirt? Where there are plenty of parking spaces but few long lines . . . and where no one is obsessed with fat grams and wrinkles?

Well, that is exactly what my husband, Eddie, and I decided to do after twenty-six years of living in Los Angeles. In 1990 we put our home up for sale in order to move to Kaua'i, Hawai'i, known as the Garden Island of the Pacific. We had clearly outgrown a lifestyle that had once seemed comfortable but now no longer nurtured us. We tried to plan carefully. We waited until our children were grown and we had enough equity in our home to support us until we were able to find work. We knew a move such as this was going to be a challenge, but we viewed it as a terrific adventure. We were joyful and excited at the thought of waking up to the beautiful azure blue ocean and watching the incomparable Hawaiian sunsets daily. As we reflect on our initial dream of simplifying our lives and moving to Kaua'i, we humorously refer to those well-intentioned ideas as Plan A.

However, as the saying goes, "the best laid plans. . . . " Soon our coveted dream began to feel more like a nightmare, as month after month the real estate market in California continued to plummet. Finally, after two and a half grueling years of meaningless open houses arranged by a succession of four real estate brokers, we sold—no, we *gave away*—our home, leaving us with almost no financial security to make this move. The equity we had counted on to provide a cushion while we got settled in our new, simpler life was no longer there. Our joyful Plan A was now a fearful "How-are-we-going-to-make-it-Plan Z"! However, with a nothing-is-going-to-stop-us-from-following-our-dream attitude, on August 31, 1992, we tearfully boarded a United Airlines DC-10, landing seven hours later in the little Lihue Airport, along with nineteen pieces of excess baggage. After leaving behind all that was familiar, supportive, and secure for most of our twenty-eight years of marriage—family, dear friends, and a thriving private practice of eighteen years—we were on Kaua'i at last.

After such an emotional time of struggling to sell our house and then pulling up roots and finally leaving, I thought I would feel elated to have arrived. I didn't. Instead I felt a great claw of fear gripping my heart as we drove to what was to be our new home in the very quiet, small town of Kekaha, located on Kaua'i's remote west side. Day by day, the enormity of the move became more real to me. This was no longer a dream, it was now a reality. We were in Paradise, but with no known means of earning a living, almost no financial resources to fall back on, and being so far from friends, family, and my spiritual roots, I wondered if I could endure the feelings of loss and fear. I truly did not know. I knew that I needed time to do nothing . . . to just be . . . to ponder what this great life change was all about.

After nine days of sleeping on the floor on an air mattress, our 267 cartons of furniture, clothing, and life essentials arrived. It was now September 10, 1992, and there I sat on the white-tiled living room floor of our two-bedroom, tin-roofed home—amidst the forest of boxes waiting to be unpacked.

Feeling tired, worn out, and overwhelmed, I suddenly found myself sobbing as I continued to unpack. "Are we crazy? What have we done?" I wondered to myself. With tears streaming down my face I said to Eddie, "I don't think I can take one more thing right now." Eddie suggested that we stop our unpacking frenzy and go out for dinner at Keoki's, one of our favorite restaurants. During dinner, the winds were blowing strong and the rain was tropically heavy. Nothing unusual for Kaua'i. Moist, balmy, and alive. We reflected on our move, the wonderful party our friends had given for us before we left, the Native American blessing ceremony given to us by many we have come to call our relatives, our children and other family members, and the hopes and dreams for an easier, different lifestyle here on Kaua'i. It was a lovely evening, and even as the winds and rain increased their intensity, I finally began to relax.

During the drive home, we noticed that the markets were unusually crowded and the gas lines very long. Not really processing what was happening, we just laughed and thought there must be some big baseball game going on for the kids. Island dwellers were very involved in their children's sports activities. But then we got to our own town and saw that the Big Save Market was still open—*and* it was very *very* crowded. We both got an ominous feeling as we recalled that earlier in the week, our friends had talked about a hurricane off the coast, which was expected to miss Kaua'i. Nothing too much to worry about at the time.

At that point we turned on the radio and heard what seemed to be unbelievable. . . . The island of Kaua'i was going to be hit by Hurricane Iniki the next afternoon (September 11) and we should prepare to evacuate to the nearest designated shelter. We were silenced by shocked disbelief. Returning home, we robotically went through the motions of trying to secure what we owned. We fastened all the windows with masking tape, locked closets, carefully stored what was treasured and breakable, and took with us only what we could carry. We called one son in California, one son in Arizona, and my parents in Nevada to tell them we would be evacuating and would call when we could. I went by the beach and offered a prayer, went back into the house, took whatever else I could put into the truck, especially our most sacred things, closed the door, and at 5:30 A.M., with the sirens blaring, we checked into the Waimea High School shelter and immediately volunteered with the Red Cross.

It all seemed unreal . . . we had just gotten to Kaua'i after a horrendous two and a half years of trying to move . . . and here we were, finally, in Paradise. Only Paradise was now being threatened by what turned out to be the most destructive storm ever to hit the Hawaiian Islands and the third most costly natural disaster in the United States per capita.

We volunteered and helped over 1,000 people check into our shelter alone. As everyone shifted into comfortable positions, we all began talking about our families, experiences, and beliefs. In Hawai'i, this is called "talking story"—and story blanketed the shelter in its

12

own form of comfort. I had lived through disasters in California, but never have I been in a place of such imminent danger where the spirit of the people outweighed the fear. It was truly a gift to experience. Everything these people owned was at great risk, yet the focus was on faith and spirit, not on panic and self-centeredness. Despite enormous overcrowding, people graciously moved to make room for one another. They reassured those who couldn't find water not to worry, for they would share what they had with them—never clinging to the fear that there wouldn't be enough for "me."

After hours of working together to create as safe a shelter as possible, it was time to close the doors. The winds had begun . . . Iniki was here in her rumbling full force. With a very human sense of curiosity, many of us peeked through the wooden louvers of the shelter, only to see trees uprooted as if they were toothpicks, church steeples toppled, roofs and homes lifted off their foundations before our eyes. And then there was one particular moment when the winds were at their strongest—227-mile-per-hour gusts—and the concrete and cinder-block building in which we were harbored seemed to be swaying. Suddenly, with a deafening power and enormous force, the overhead steel and wooden louvers blew out, scattering debris everywhere. Moving quickly, everyone began to overturn huge cafeteria tables and benches to hide under for protection from the flying debris. Looking at the heaviness of those tables today, I don't know where my strength came from at the time. I could hear Eddie's voice through the roaring sound of the wind, calling for me to be careful and *get down*. For some unexplainable reason I was not concerned about getting hit by flying objects—things were happening too fast.

Eddie and I huddled together under one of the tables as the winds of Iniki continued with her pounding force. It was during this breath-holding moment that tears came to the eyes of my husband, as he kept repeating in a somewhat mantra-like monotone fashion, "I know we've lost everything . . . I know we've lost everything" . . . and it was also in that tender moment of pain and fear over what seemed to be certain loss that a dream I had just before our move flashed through my mind like a bolt of unexpected lightning electrifying my fear-darkened inner-sky of thought. While remaining crouched under one of the overturned lunchroom tables and the thunderous noise of the wind continuing its pounding force, I decided to share this illuminating dream with Eddie.

I told him that about two months before moving to Kaua'i, fear began to ripple through my body on a daily basis. My inner dialogue was going wild with thoughts such as "Am I crazy to give up everything that I know that has been safe and familiar? Am I nuts to move away from everyone I love, give up my home of twenty-six years, to move to a place we have only visited but never lived in? Where neither of us will have jobs or known sources of income?" These and other questions of fear began to surface more and more each day as the time for the move grew closer.

One night as I was restlessly lying in bed, I prayed for a dream that would help me through this time of fear. I felt like I was shaking the tree of faith for help . . . for faith in the decision to change the way we were living, to allow a possibility for new growth of self and soul. Finally, after a seemingly endless time of tossing and turning, I entered the Place of the Dreamtime and I was presented with the following gift.

I am walking toward a large field, perhaps one where a Native American Ceremony such as a Pow-Wow has just taken place. Coming towards me are a man and a woman. The woman is carrying a large bird cradled in her arms—only the tail feathers are showing, as the head is tucked under her arm. The man is carrying a large gray and white bird with a long neck and beautiful feathers. I recognized the woman's bird as an owl. I commented on how beautiful her bird was and said that the owl is a sacred bird in Hawai'i. I then went over to the man and said, "Oh, that's a medicine bird—it's very beautiful. You know, I go to these ceremonies and I would really like to have some feathers for a giveaway to my relatives. So whenever you have extra feathers to spare, I would sure appreciate them."

The tall, kind man then moved closer and gently, with graceful, ballet-like hand movements, turned the bird over, reached underneath it, and held out two handfuls of feathers. Looking softly into my eyes he said, "Yes, this is a medicine bird. Now hold out your hands." I did as the man asked, extending both of my hands. He then placed the feathers on the palms of my hands and said, "Here, they are called Faith, *and you have all that you need."*

When I awoke, my hands were extended as I lay in bed and I found myself gently moving my fingers, as if caressing the feathers placed there. I remained in bed for over an hour, thinking about what that dream meant to me. I realized that the man and the woman were messengers of both the feminine and masculine aspects of God. As I pondered their message, I believe it was telling me that while there were still many unknowns regarding the move for me to face, I was also being given the greatest medicine for confronting my fears, which was faith . . . faith in the form of the feathers. I remember feeling a deep sense of comfort and relief as I continued to reflect on the message of the dream.

After I finished telling Eddie about my dream, I noticed that he had extended his hands as if he, too, had received the feathers of faith in this moment of intense fear.

It was many hours until all was quiet once again. Together we ate, talked story, and slept on the floor, benches, and tables in the shelter until morning, when it was announced that it would be safe to go home.

Driving slowly through the hurricane-ravaged streets, we picked our way through downed power lines, destroyed homes, overturned cars, and toppled trees. As we rounded the corner to our street, which faced the ocean where waves had reached a reported thirty feet, my husband stopped the truck for a moment in fear of what we might see just ahead. Sharing in that same human moment of fear of what might have been lost . . . the message of my dream streamed through my consciousness as powerfully as the sun shines its rays through the windows of the clouds. I then reminded Eddie of the dream and its message that we have all that we need to confront our fears lying within the palms of our hands . . . *faith*. Once again the message of faith outshined the grip of fear.

As we approached, we saw that our roof had blown off, there were many trees downed, and there were dead fish and debris strewn every-where . . . but our home? . . . It was miraculously standing! Our little tin-roofed, single-walled, glass-louver-windowed home, standing just a few hundred feet from the powerful ocean, had survived the most ferocious storm to hit the Hawaiian Islands. How or why? I cannot answer such questions. I only know that it did.

What have I learned over the years from this experience? While I am still pondering that question for myself, I can tell you what I have learned thus far, and it is this: All of us live through hurricanes in one form or another. And that there are many kinds of shelter in which we can seek safety from these personal storms. However, the most powerful shelter of all is built within the human Soul. It is called *faith*.

Each day as new challenges present themselves to me, and I feel the weight of fear beginning to settle heavily on my chest, I remember what the tall, kind man in my dream said to me, and I hold out my hands and feel the feathers of faith placed there . . . and I am reminded that I truly have all that I need.

Steppingstone One

THE DREAMING POT

"Man is never alone. Acknowledged or unacknowledged, that which dreams through him is always there to support him from within."

—Laurens van der Post[3]

Oftentimes in the face of trauma, pain, and fear, the visions of our dreams and sense of identity can get shrouded in an all-encompassing veil of darkness. It is at these life-challenging times that the symbols in our dreams must be reawakened and brought forward to help us manage and heal from the struggles that temporarily blind us to the possibilities, solutions, and simple joys of life.

The idea of Dreaming Pots came to me several years ago while I was visiting one of my favorite spots in Arizona—the Heard Museum. This Native American museum is filled with art, stories, and experiences that touch the heart, educate the mind, and embrace the spirit.

As I was enjoying my time wandering through the museum, I came upon a pottery exhibit from the ancient Mimbres tribe, which provides a unique window into the prehistoric life and cosmology of the people. The pottery bowls were distinctively painted with symbolic designs that told the story of everyday life and ceremonies. What sparked my attention most were the holes that were in the bottom of each bowl. Although little is known about the specifics of the bowls, it is known that they were placed in the burial site when a person died. One story that is hypothesized is that the bowls were placed in the burial site to bring good spirits to those who had died and the holes allowed the departed spirit to travel freely and unconstrained. Another part of the story was that the holes also allowed negativity to be released and not held as the person made his or her journey to the spirit world.

The experience of hearing the story and seeing the pottery stayed with me long after I left the museum. That night, as I lay in bed I thought to myself, "This is wonderful. But how can we use the idea of pots such as these in life, without having to wait for death?" I wanted to be able to use them personally, as well as with the children, families, and individuals with whom I worked . . . with those whose dreams were dimmed by the traumas of life.

And so I closed my eyes, took a deep breath, and reviewed the story in my mind. It then came to me. I began to think of death as a form of sleep . . . and when we sleep, we dream. And so the idea of dreaming came into my mind. Excitedly I thought, "We can make Dreaming Pots."

Not being a potter, I thought of using ready-made clay pots with the holes already in the bottom, that can easily be purchased for a very nominal fee from a flower nursery. I wanted to use clay because that is the material of the earth. The next day I bought several pots, as well as beads, feathers, and paint to decorate them. After unloading the boxes of supplies in my office, I sat down on a small wooden stool by my art table, took out one of the pots, closed my eyes, took a deep breath, and let the symbols of my dreams stream forth. When I was ready, I opened my eyes and began to decorate the pot with those symbols. I do not remember exactly how long I sat there, but I do remember the sense of relaxation and enjoyment I was experiencing.

Since that time, Dreaming Pots have become a powerful healing tool in my personal life and work. To date, the children and families of Kaua'i have made more than four hundred dreaming pots. This activity was particularly meaningful for the children because many of their homes had been destroyed in the hurricane, and they were sleeping on the floor in the homes of others or in tents. They were afraid to go to sleep and experienced many nightmares. By making their own Dreaming Pots, the children could put them by their sleeping places and be reminded of their good dreams. It gave them something tangible to focus upon that brought comfort and a sense of inner control.

And so I invite you to create your own Dreaming Pot, and enjoy discovering a reconnection to your dreams, aspirations, and visions. Remember, "A dream is a wish your heart makes. . . ."

Making Your Own Dreaming Pot

This steppingstone exercise is designed to help you reconnect to those dreams that bring joy, empowerment, and self-appreciation. You can create your own Dreaming Pot in two ways:

(1) by following the instructions for making a "Hands-On" version, using an actual clay pot, paint, and other supplies of art and nature, or (2) by drawing an image of your Dreaming Pot using the page provided in this book.

THE HANDS-ON VERSION

1. Use a small clay pot with a hole in the bottom, which can be purchased at a nursery. (Of course, if you are a potter, you can make your own.) You will also need acrylic paints of various colors of your choice, paint brushes, and anything else you might want to include on your pot, such as small rocks, shells, flowers, sand, earth, and so on.

2. Find a comfortable place in which to work. Hold the pot in your hands, close your eyes, take a few slow deep breaths, inhaling through your nose and exhaling through your mouth, and, in a sense, "introduce" yourself to the pot. I know this may seem strange, but remember you are making a connection with it, as if you were meeting someone special for the first time. For example, I hold the pot in my hands and feel all parts of it with my fingers and palms. I say in my mind, "Hello, I am Joyce and I have come here to share my dreams."

   Think this is weird stuff? Well, remember, pilots often name and talk to their planes . . . those who work with computers often have names for them . . . many of us name our cars . . . not to mention golfers who talk to their clubs! This is no different.

3. Now allow images and symbols from your good dreams, aspirations, and visions to come to your mind. When the images are clear, take another slow breath, open your eyes, and begin creating your Dreaming Pot with the art supplies you have gathered.

   Option: Each night draw a picture of what you want in your life right now. Place the finished drawing in the pot by your bed and enjoy the dreams brought to you while you sleep. In the morning you can take the picture out of the pot and put it in an album, thereby creating a Dreaming Pot journal.

The Drawn Version

Apply these same steps to the drawing of your Dreaming Pot on the following page. The only change is to imagine holding the pot in your hands before you begin to draw it. All else remains the same. As Shakespeare said, "We are such stuff as dreams are made on." Let the symbols of your dreams emerge with breath and vision, thereby providing you with another steppingstone for you to walk upon on your journeys of life.

My Dreaming Pot

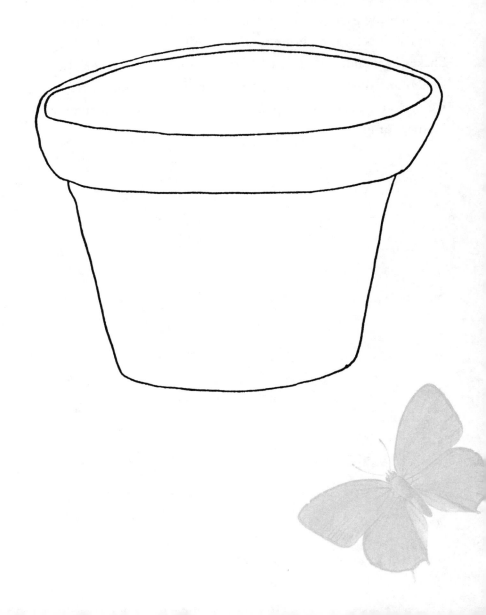

CHAPTER TWO

God Speaks Even in Big Save Market

*"Your sacred space is where you
can find yourself again and again."*

—Joseph Campbell[4]

om Kippur is one of the most sacred holidays for the Jewish People . . . my tribe. Beginning at sundown, when the holiday begins, Jewish people all over the world fast for twenty-four hours . . . no food, no water. It is a time of prayer, sacrifice, and atonement, of taking the time to look inward at how you have treated yourself and others over the past year. It is a time to wipe the slate clean, so to speak, and begin the Jewish New Year with a cleansed sense of self and a reconnection to faith.

I remember growing up in the Bronx with my Bubbie (the Yiddish word for grandmother) and my mother, Rose, in our little one-bedroom apartment, feeling the excitement coupled with the seriousness of the holiday. As sundown approached, the neighborhood was literally shut down in respect. My Bubbie had already prepared the meal for the breaking of the fast. Most of the Jewish community went to synagogue and stayed all day in prayer. I went at times, but there were times I couldn't go, because my Bubbie and my mother weren't able to go. I remember asking, "Bubbie, don't we have to go to synagogue to pray?" This little woman, standing all of four feet ten inches tall, would answer me in Yiddish, "*Joyce-ala*, where you stand, you pray."

At that young age of five or six, I didn't know what her words meant . . . "Where you stand, you pray." Little did I know that, some forty-five years later, I would finally understand my Bubbie's words.

It was September 14, 1994, the Jewish year of 5755, around 4:15 P.M. I had just finished working with my clients for the day and went to the Big Save Market in our neighborhood to pick up some last-minute food for that evening's holiday meal and for the breaking of the fast the next day. This was to be our third year celebrating this sacred holiday in Kaua'i, without the gift of loving relatives and friends. For twenty-eight years while living in Los Angeles, our home on holidays was always filled to the brim with those whom we called "family," no matter what their religion. I cooked for days ahead of time, preparing traditional foods such as gefilte fish, chopped liver, and, of course, the food for the soul, chicken soup and matzoh balls. Those who came brought their own goodies to share with all who were present.

On this night, the eve of Yom Kippur, my husband had to work. Eddie would be with me the following day and evening, to pray and break the fast together, but I was going to be alone on this sacred evening known as Kol Nidre.

I had already begun to evaluate my time living in Kaua'i. It had been two years since our move, two years since Hurricane Iniki had struck. The first time we celebrated Yom Kippur on Kaua'i was right after the hurricane, and instead of the traditional foods to break the fast, we used canned corn and Spam. I had also found a small box of raisins and a package of noodles at the time, along with a few eggs, and managed to cook a kugel (a sort of pie-type pudding) on a small, round barbecue. I shared it with the volunteers with whom we had been working at the Waimea Neighborhood Center and told them about this sacred holiday of Yom Kippur. It was truly a time of prayer, reflection, and gratefulness.

Now some two years later, I thought that, surely by this time, my life would be in order, my path clear. No such luck. Things were just as uncertain, just as unpredictable, as they had been since our decision to move in 1990. With government grants for child and family services being drastically cut, my professional license of two decades not honored in the state of Hawai'i, as well as my professional experience as a trainer in the field of mental health not being utilized, I wondered how I would earn a living.

Even my sense of creativity had vanished. While working on this book, every word that I wrote seemed to fall apart as it was being written. My thoughts jumped around like the little jumping beans I used to hold in the palms of my hands as a child. I was feeling lonely and disconnected from my spiritual sources—not just my community of Jewish friends and relatives, but from those Native American people whom I called relatives as well. I deeply missed sharing the rituals and ceremonies that were part of our lives for so many years.

Needless to say, this was a time of great uncertainty . . . and as often happens, uncertainty brings a sense of fear.

So there I was on the eve of Yom Kippur, wandering the isles of Big Save Market in the little town of Waimea, contemplating the meaning of my life. Suddenly, while standing in the aisle between the frozen food and aluminum foil, I heard the gentle Southern voice of Abraham, a tall, slender African-American man in his early eighties. I had come to know Abraham from my work at the Waimea Neighborhood Center. He would stop in my office from time to time and we would just enjoy "talking story," as they say in Hawai'i. Abraham is a basket weaver.

"Hello, Joyce," Abraham greeted me. His twinkling eyes and smile lit up the aisle. "I've been looking for you. Have you been away?" he asked. "No," I replied, "I've just changed my hours a bit." At that point, Abraham opened a plastic bag he was holding, reached inside and said, "I have been looking for you because I have a gift for you." With that, he handed me a palm-sized, round straw basket with a delicately woven lid on it. "Here," he said. "I made this for you." Graciously, I extended my hand to receive this special gift, smiled, and gave Abraham a great big thank-you hug.

There I stood in the middle of Big Save Market, between the frozen food and aluminum foil, holding this treasure made and given by *Abraham*. We finished our conversation and said our farewells for the day. I carefully placed the basket in the top shelf of my cart and finished my shopping. At this time I was unaware of a deeper significance to this meeting with Abraham and his gift beyond the fact that I adored our friendship and was deeply grateful for his gift.

I went home and put the basket on the writing desk in my small, very cluttered office. Abraham's gift seemed to be talking to me, but I couldn't quite make out its message. Then, while on the phone with a very dear friend, talking about this chapter on fear and faith, I glanced at the basket and began to chuckle. "What are you laughing about, Joyce?" she questioned. "Oh, my," I blurted out, "God speaks even in Big Save Market, between the frozen food and aluminum foil!" I went on to tell my friend about how I was feeling earlier that day . . . lonely, confused, and worried . . . when I met *Abraham* and received his gift.

"This holiday is about *faith*," I continued. "God speaks to *Abraham* and asks him to sacrifice his first-born son to prove his commitment to God. Abraham does as God asks and prepares his precious son Isaac for the sacrifice. But just as he is about to kill him, God speaks by providing a sacrificial ram for Abraham to use in his son's place. It was a true test of faith. So there I was on Yom Kippur eve, feeling confused, worried, and lonely, feeling like I had sacrificed everything and questioning for what, when God spoke again through a man named Abraham. In a sense I heard God say, 'Have faith Joyce, I have not forgotten you . . . Take this gift as a reminder' . . . Get it! *Abraham . . . Yom Kippur . . . sacrifice . . . a test of faith . . . a gift!*" After a few moments of reflective silence, we both laughed at the way in which spiritual teachings present themselves at the most unexpected times.

Earlier that day, I had planned to go into town to a prayer service being held some forty miles from my house. However, in the quiet peacefulness of this special night, I realized that prayers are not something you begin by opening a book or by sitting in a room. Prayers are something you live. I remembered the words of my Bubbie when she would say to me, "*Joyce-ala*, where you stand, you pray." I realized that I had been praying all evening.

How did my feelings change from worry, confusion, and gnawing disconnectedness to those of relatedness, gratefulness, and appreciation? What was the magic that created this change? Reflecting back, the magic was in that one suspended moment in time when Abraham said, "Here, I made this gift for you," and handed me the basket. In my time of confusion and doubt about my newly risked direction in life . . . fearful whether or not we had made the right decision to move . . . I had received another "feather of faith," a faith contained in every strand of straw which Abraham had woven into this gift.

Yes, God speaks even in Big Save Market, between the frozen food and aluminum foil . . . and Yes, Bubbie, you were right, "Where you stand, you pray."

Steppingstone Two

PRAYERFULNESS

*"Prayer is a voice from the heart that
goes directly to the tongue, it's a heartsong."*

—Carl Hammerschlag, M.D.[5]

Have you ever asked yourself what prayer means to you? Does it mean going to a church, temple, mosque, or some other special place of worship? Does it mean reading a passage from a bible, or perhaps just sitting down under a tree, by a river, or taking a walk in the park and just talking to God, your Higher Power, Mother, Jesus, Adonai, Allah, Buddha, Jehovah, angels, or whomever or whatever you may call the intercessor of spirit in your life? Perhaps in our busy days of work, family, or school we forget to take time out to pray . . . to connect to something greater than ourselves. In his book *Healing Words: The Power of Prayer and the Practice of Medicine,*[6] Dr. Larry Dossey writes that some people "do not pray in any conventional sense, but live with a deeply interiorized sense of the sacred. Theirs

29

could be called a spirit of prayerfulness, a sense of simply being attuned or aligned with 'something higher'." Perhaps my Bubbie fits into this latter group.

This steppingstone is meant to help you traverse the rivers of prayer and to help you recognize a "spirit of prayerfulness" in your everyday life.

- First find a quiet place and ask yourself,

  "What do prayer and prayerfulness mean to me?"
- Next ask yourself,

  "Where do I pray?" "Where am I prayerful?"
- Now ask yourself,

  "When do I pray?" "When am I prayerful?"
- Finally, take time out each day to say a prayer of gratitude, honor your Beingness and remember, "Where you stand, you pray."

CHAPTER THREE

Dragons of Fear

*"Fear is a reminder to take a deep breath and
let go into the present moment where the love of the
Universe is a constant support."*

—Joan Borysenko, Ph.D.[7]

Slaying dragons is not a new concept in mythology. Not all cultures see dragons as monsters to be feared. In the Chinese culture dragons are seen as giving us glorious gifts. However, our Western tales tell us that dragons hold us captive in the grips of their threatening fire, ultimately rendering us unable to breathe easily or walk freely. It is this Western view of the dragon I speak about in this chapter. Dragons are a symbol of our fear and our sword is one of faith and courage.

I remember listening to a Bill Moyers interview with Joseph Campbell when they were discussing this very subject of heroes and the act of slaying dragons. Mr. Moyers asked, in essence, "Aren't we all heroes in a way?" Joseph Campbell's reply surprised me because he said that we were not all heroes. When an ordinary person knows that there is a dragon in the cave, he or she won't pick up the sword to slay it. A hero is the person who has the courage to pick up the sword, walk into the cave, and confront the dragon.

When I began writing this book, a woman I had known for some ten years came to mind. Her name is Grace, a true heroine in her own healing journey . . . a woman who was valiant enough to pick up her sword of faith, walk into her cave, and symbolically slay a fire-breathing dragon of fear that had plagued her life for many years. It is my hope that her story will empower you to confront your own dragons with a sword of courage and faith. With her loving permission I share her story.

Little six-year-old Grace played outside of the church, excitedly awaiting her First Holy Communion. However, her excitement was quickly crushed when she entered the confessional. It was there that Grace was first abused by her priest. Her young voice of prayer became silenced in a tomb of fear: The priest threatened that if she told anyone, he would hurt her and her family.

His sexual abuse and violent threats continued until Grace was in her preteen years. Even if she had decided to risk his threats and speak out on her own behalf, who would have believed the child-voice of little Grace above the God-voice of a priest? Grace's belief was "no one," and so she kept her silence guarded within her soul for many years, until she was well into adulthood . . . until one day a "hidden angel" brought her into therapy. Many of us come into therapy asking for help in one area of our lives, not aware that this *problem* is really a hidden angel in disguise, directing our paths towards a deeper healing.

Grace first came to see me for hypnosis to help her stop smoking. Initially Grace talked about her sincere desire to stop smoking. Her reasons were clear: She wanted to smell better, she was tired of being an outcast in society's changing nonsmoking environment, and she wanted to live longer. All of her reasons made perfect sense, yet soon after we started working together, it became clear that Grace wasn't ready to stop smoking. She realized that her habit served a very valuable purpose in her life, for which she hadn't been able to find a replacement. Smoking was her friend in her greatest times of loneliness. It also helped to keep her from speaking up. Her belief was that she talked too much and really had nothing to say. Grace's smoking was her "hidden angel."

Grace had a unique gift with words; she spoke in metaphor almost all of the time. She had the ability to see all of life in story and art. But often this poetic gift felt more like a curse, because it separated her from the outside world, which relied on straightforward communication styles. Grace rarely engaged in a conversation that had a recognizable through-line. This was frustrating for her and for those who tried to relate to her; she often felt misunderstood and others felt the same.

After many months of working together, Grace realized that she didn't want to stop smoking, but she did want to continue with her therapy. I suggested that she join a women's group I ran on Wednesday evenings. Grace expressed great fear of joining a group and not being accepted. I told her that the women in this group all came from different backgrounds and were dealing with different issues in their lives. What brought them together was their uniqueness. Their area of commonality was being women in a society that still largely devalued them.

Grace decided to take the risk and join the group. She diligently strove to express herself clearly, but following her train of thought remained ever difficult. The other group members were supportive but at times could not suppress their impatience with her ramblings. I often acted as a translator; woven within the tangled threads of Grace's metaphorical speech, I knew she was trying to relate in the best way she knew how, and also that she was trying to tell us something important about her life. However, at this time, I still did not know what that "something" was . . . until an event in my life ended up having wonderful repercussions for Grace and the group as a whole.

In March of 1987, I went to Arizona for a spiritual weekend retreat presented by The Turtle Island Project, a nonprofit organization dedicated to sharing a participatory vision of healing, research, educaton, and service. Co-led by psychiatrist and co-founder Dr. Carl Hammerschlag, facilitators Mona Polacca from the Hopi/Havasupai tribe, Nelson Fernandez from the Mohave tribe, and Dr. John Koriath, a neurophysiologist, the weekend combined mind-body healing philosophies along with sacred Native American ceremonies and teachings such as a sweat lodge, talking circles, vision walk, and mask-making. When I returned, the women in the group were eager to hear all about it. At that point in time, I was so pierced by the experience that I wasn't quite ready to share what I had learned. The best description of my feelings was as "numinous," meaning that the experiences had a deeply spiritual and mystical effect on me, unexplainable in words. These ceremonies were not techniques to get us to express ourselves, or contrived to get us to change in some way, as is the case with approaches in psychotherapy. Instead these were ancient teachings to help put us "in relation" to the magic of life with all of its challenges and blessings. Because the teachings were also very sacred to Native American people, as Baptism is to Christianity and the Bar or Bat Mitzvah is to Judaism, I wasn't sure what I could or couldn't share. But after a time of careful consideration and talking with Mona I began to share what I learned . . . especially in relation to the honoring of women . . . something I felt that was greatly lacking in our non-Native society.

Now with encouragement and permission from my teachers, I began each group by lighting sage, as I had learned to do on the retreat. Many Native American people use sage for purification in ceremonies and rituals. The fragrant smoke helped to bring a sense of the Sacred into the room. Instead of an ordinary psychotherapy group where women simply talked about their feelings and experiences, we were creating an atmosphere of ritual and ceremony, a place where the opening into the spiritual perspectives of healing were welcomed. Little did I realize at the time that the lighting of the sage would provide an opening into the darkness that still shrouded Grace's life.

Grace requested a private session, and it was in that session that she finally chose to reveal the secret she had been harboring deep within the safety of her soul. She told me that it was the smell of the sage that reminded her of the church in which her precious innocence had been violated. Grace's foundation of faith had been shattered in the very sanctuary that was supposed to protect and nurture her young Soul. She had kept her secret until she could keep it no longer.

Grace said that since all of the abuse started in the confessional box, she would tell her story as if she were confessing. In her words, "This time it is a confession of healing" instead of a confession of shame. She said that, rather than just give an account of the "bad things" the priest had done to her, she would "confess" what she believed she had done that was bad. Grace continued to struggle to find words to describe how she had felt as a child.

To ensure her silence, the priest had threatened her life and the safety of her sisters. As a consequence, Grace remained silent as his assaults continued throughout her preteen years. Her life became a tormented prison of fear, shame, and secrecy. As this vaulted doorway to Grace's prison finally began to open, I pondered and reflected on the depth of her wounding and how best to help her find healing for her torment. I decided to invite her to a women's retreat similar to the retreat I had previously attended, only this one was for women only. I was co-leading the weekend with Mona and felt it would be a soul-nurturing experience for Grace. Bravely, Grace decided to come to our Women's Healing Journey retreat in March of 1988, along with other women from our group.

There she confronted her lifelong fears that had linked rituals and ceremonies with trauma and abuse. Through experiences like the sweat lodge, talking circle, and a woman's honoring ceremony, Grace began to dismantle her cloak of terror and allow herself a glimpse into the face of faith.

The culmination of Grace's weekend experience, and her support in group and individual counseling, was her decision to confront her fears directly. She enlisted my help in locating the priest. First she contacted the archdiocese and told her story. She received a loving and supportive letter from the Bishop in her home state, who also gave her information about the priest's location. The Bishop told her that the man was no longer a priest and he was now married and living in another state. She then proceeded to write to him. I told her she could use my office as a return address. She did.

Grace then decided that writing wasn't enough and she wanted to confront him, face to face. Using a Jane Doe alias, Grace called him and told him that she was writing an article on priests from her hometown who had left the priesthood and wanted to interview him. He agreed. With all of her savings, Grace flew to confront the man who had ravaged her childhood years. Grace said she sat parked outside of his home for what seemed like hours, but was really only a few minutes, before she could muster the courage to open the car door and walk up to his house. Her feet felt hot and a voice in her head said, "I don't need to do this . . . He could kill me." Just as powerfully, another voice countered, "You need to see him NOW." She recalls, "I had to remember all the positive stuff I learned in therapy to help me."

Mustering all of her courage, Grace knocked on his door. After so many years of grueling shame and pain, she now stood face to face with her abuser. He looked shriveled and gray, no longer scary-looking. He invited her into his living room, which looked like a shrine to himself. There were pictures of him with the Pope as well as with other respected religious leaders. There were also pictures of him and his family. When Grace saw the many pictures of the little girls in his family, a sickening feeling came over her as she flashed on what he might have done to them. At that moment, she had to control every emotion in her body to restrain herself from attacking him. He bragged that he was still very active with the church, and then, perhaps in a moment of recognition, he asked her if she knew a girl named *Grace*. Grace stood up and looked him directly in his eyes and said, "I know her better than you." Grace says that at the point when she rose to stand and face him, she knew that, from then on, she would be able to stand up for anything in her life.

Remaining standing, Grace went on to "confess" to him all the horrible things that priest had done to the little girl, Grace. She continued to speak in the third person. She used the word *confess* because she knew that a priest—even a former one—was bound by confidentiality. She no longer wanted to carry the secret. It was time to make him carry it.

He responded by saying that he had taught Grace a lot about God, and that as a priest, he had done this for her own good. His words twisted in the air. No longer a little girl being threatened to keep a secret, Grace was well aware of his attempted manipulations. She retorted, "It *wasn't* a teaching . . . it was *not* about God . . . It *is* about *hurt.*"

Grace said she needed no more "details." The meeting, for her, was about confronting her demons, and she had done so. Later that night, while in her hotel room, she felt like a little child . . . singing, eating lots of junk food, staying up as late as she wanted. Perhaps this was a spontaneous way of celebrating that her inner child was finally set free from the shame and fear that had imprisoned her for what appeared to be a life sentence. The next morning she was on the plane on her way back home to Los Angeles. She had survived her greatest fear . . . that he would get her again.

Since then, Grace has gone back to school, become a registered art therapist, and is working on a book of her own. Does Grace still have fears? Yes, but fear no longer controls her every waking moment. The fear has been replaced by faith. When I asked Grace for her definition of faith, after a lingering pause, she replied, "Faith is doing stuff anyway." The answer of a true heroine.

Steppingstone Three

INNER RESOURCE DRAWINGS

*"I saw art as a magic mirror making
visible what is invisible in us and the life of our time."*

—Laurens van der Post[8]

 ach of us has dragons that keep us from enjoying life fully. Whether it is physical pain from an illness or emotional pain such as fear, wouldn't it be wonderful to have a magic wand of sorts that could *whoosh-away* problems and worrisome feelings with a simple wave of the wrist? I think it would. "If I could just get a better handle on the problem, I would be able to find the solution . . . I feel lost, I just can't find an answer" are some of the feelings expressed while we search for the perfect answers. Usually we try to talk it out with a friend, colleague, or professional counselor. Sometimes just talking it out is enough, but oftentimes we go round and round as if chasing our own tails for the solutions . . . we analyze, analyze, analyze until our brains feel like they're going to explode. Sometimes it is just time to stop the jabber and find other avenues that will lead us to the much-sought-after solutions.

One of the ways I have found to open the pathways to solutions is to use what Dr. Richard Crowley and I call "Inner Resource Drawings." In our book *Therapeutic Metaphors for Children and the Child Within*,[9] we give a number of case examples of how we use this drawing approach in our work with children to facilitate healing physical and emotional pain, as well as to increase self-esteem. We discovered that Inner Resource Drawings help our clients in two ways: they give them a tool to gain control over a pain or over their emotional responses to a problem; and they also help them discover a "healing bridge" that leads them from the problem to the solution.

The beauty of Inner Resource Drawings is that they work as steppingstones to help each person discover his or her own personal images and symbols that represent not only the problem, but also the solution and the unconscious medicine. In other words, what sets this drawing approach apart from others is that it doesn't stop at just identifying a problem; it brings forth the vision of a solution. And vision is what we need when we are trapped in the grip of nagging problems.

For example, there was the time I was visiting eight-year-old Suzie, who was in the hospital for tests to determine the cause of sharp pains she was experiencing in the area of her kidneys. Suzie is the daughter of one of my dearest friends and also like a niece to me. As we visited, I noticed Suzie wincing. I asked her what was wrong and with a tender, shaky voice Suzie said, "It hurts real bad here," pointing to her side. I then asked her if she had crayons, markers, and paper. She said yes and gestured over to her nightstand on which there were a colorful spiraled notebook and some markers. I handed her the notebook and markers and asked her if she would play a little with me. Even through her pain, the word *play* brought a smile to her face. "Sure," she replied. I then asked her to close her eyes, take a deep breath, and imagine seeing what the pain "looks" like. I told her that when she had the picture in her mind, she was to open her eyes and draw it. Without hesitation, Suzie did as suggested. When she opened her eyes, she eagerly began drawing her pain.

Next I asked Suzie to draw a picture of "what the pain would look like all better." She began drawing her second picture with barely a slight pause. While she was drawing this picture, it was clear that her face was more relaxed than before we began drawing.

Finally I asked Suzie to take a third piece of paper and draw "what would help change picture one into picture two." Suzie immediately started to draw her third picture, which I call the unconscious medicine or metaphorical bridge. Spontaneously, Suzie turned to her mother, who was in the room, and said, "The pain doesn't hurt so much." She took a pen and wrote "My Pain Getting Better Book"[10] on the cover. Suzie continued drawing in her book the whole time she remained in the hospital. Each of her pictures had a similar theme of music in the third picture. This let us know that Suzie's inner resource for healing— her unconscious medicine, her healing bridge—had to do with music.

Another experience was with twenty-two-year-old Jennifer, a prelaw student who was referred to me because of acute panic attacks. Her heart would beat rapidly, she would become sweaty and unable to catch her breath. She was rushed to the emergency hospital quite regularly, only to have physical problems ruled out. This situation was causing increasing difficulty for her, because she couldn't study or remain in a classroom without wanting to run outside. Jennifer was seen by a physician and was given antianxiety medication, which was not working. Her attacks were increasing and her fears were becoming stronger.

In our first session I gave Jennifer three sheets of paper and asked her to draw a picture of the anxiety on one of the papers. She immediately picked up a black marker and began drawing. I then gave her a second paper and asked her to draw what the anxiety would look like when it was all better. Without hesitation she picked up the red marker and began drawing. After she was satisfied with her second "all better" picture, I asked her to draw what would change picture one into picture two. Jennifer reached for the yellow marker and immediately began drawing a picture resembling a feminine figure in a relaxed position. I asked Jennifer to look at picture one and notice what she felt. She crinkled her nose and said, "Yuk!" I then asked her to hold up her second picture and describe what she noticed. She held it for a moment or two, gave a deep sigh, and smiled. Next I asked her to hold up her third picture and repeated the instructions. She continued smiling and said, "I like looking at it."

I did not tell Jennifer what colors to choose, nor did I analyze any part of her drawings. The point was to give Jennifer a valuable tool to help her gain control over the devouring feeling of fear that came over her. Jennifer decided to carry a colorfully bound, blank notebook in her purse, and whenever she started to experience the slightest sensation of an attack coming on, she would repeat these three steps. Each time she used the same colors to depict her problem, solution, and unconscious medicine . . . and each time her third picture was one of a feminine figure in a relaxed, yoga-like position. Inner Resource Drawings became a valuable tool in Jennifer's therapy that helped her gain control over her imprisoning anxiety. Ultimately, her healing generalized to her ability to meet the difficult challenges of law school and new relationships. She graduated with honors and is now a practicing attorney.

Eagle Vision

You may be saying to yourself, "Great, but what does that have to do with my situation? How does and why would drawing help me with my feelings of fear and helplessness? I'm not a kid, I don't have time for such nonsense. I need solutions NOW!" Well, rather than delving into the clinical explanations as to *why* drawing is healing, let's "walk the talk" and learn how.

- First, get some markers, crayons, or drawing pencils.
- Next, choose a fear or a problem you'd like to confront. Close your eyes and take a few deep breaths to clear your mind and relax your body, and let an image of your fear/problem come to mind. Notice its color, shape, size.
- When you have that image, open your eyes and draw it on the page in this book entitled: *My Problem.*
- On the next page, *My All-Better Picture*, draw how **that** picture (the problem/fear) **looks** feeling "all better."
- Finally, on the third page, *My Healing Bridge*, draw a symbol of what will change picture one into picture two, perhaps asking yourself where in your life you have had that "all better" feeling.

This is an important point: notice I didn't say "draw how *you are feeling*" or draw what *you think* would change picture one to picture two. That's because it is important to separate from the problem so that you can gain a greater perspective. Gaining a greater perspective is the difference between seeing with the eyes of a mouse and seeing with the eyes of an eagle. To gain mastery over our problems, we must see with the eyes of an eagle, for the eagle has the ability to fly the highest and see in all directions. And then, when it finds just what it needs, with purpose and strength the eagle focuses in and secures nourishment for itself and its young. The mouse only sees what is in front of its nose and often misses the vast choices up ahead.

Our goal is to learn *how* to broaden our perspective, so that we can expand our choices when our vision is limited by the blinders of fear, anger, or self-doubt . . . when our inner resources are being blocked by our fire-breathing dragons of fear and life's challenges. Inner Resource Drawings can be a valuable tool in that quest.

Now take a moment and look at each of your drawings *one at a time* and notice what you experience in your body . . . any new sensations, breathing changes, warmth or coolness, heart-rate changes. While gazing at the first picture many people say that they have the desire to rip it up and throw it away. The second and third pictures often evoke a smile, a gentle sigh, or a sense of relaxation. Yet each of us is different and it is important to respect our own unique response.

Variations on Inner Resource Drawings

I am often asked, "Why draw the third picture? Isn't the 'all-better' picture enough?" In some cases it is. For children as young as two years old, the all-better picture is quite effective. After Hurricane Iniki I taught many parents how to use this approach to help their preschool children with the fears that lingered after the storm. It was not uncommon for these children to experience nightmares and generalized fear when going to sleep or whenever the winds began to blow strong again in normal tropical fashion. During one of our Parent Talk-Story Groups, Peggy, the mother of three-year-old twin girls, shared her concerns about her daughters' fears. I suggested that each time the girls said they were afraid, Peggy should suggest that they draw how the afraid feeling looks on one page, followed by "how the afraid feeling would look feeling all better" on a second page. Peggy would hang their all-better pictures near their beds and teach the girls the Magic Happy Breath[11] technique (a child's version of the Mini-Mind Vacation exercise mentioned in Steppingstone

Twelve), letting them gaze at their picture as they breathed comfortably before falling asleep.

Peggy came back the following week and said that both of her daughters had painted both pictures and that afterwards, the girls began to sleep through the night and became noticeably less clingy. Peggy continued with these drawings each time the girls became fearful, along with offering them plenty of cuddling and reassurance.

Of course, it is perfectly normal to be fearful after a traumatic event. Still, it is important to find the tools that can help us cope and heal from such experiences. Inner Resource Drawings is a tool, a Steppingstone, for you to take along on your path of healing and empowerment.

My Problem

My All-Better Feeling

My Healing Bridge

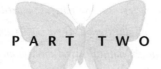

Lessons Learned from the Natural World

"Nature is a collection of systems, forces, flows,
pulses, and heartbeats— all woven together into a
tapestry of pure magic, just like each person.
You can understand real magic only
by experiencing it."

—James A. Swain[1]

"*I used to know an old man who would walk by any cornfield and hear the corn singing.*" *This gentle quote opens the wonderful children's book* The Other Way to Listen.[2] *Through story and illustration, Byrd Baylor and Peter Parnall take us on a journey of relationship with the natural world through an old man and a young boy. The philosophy that we can talk with nature and learn important lessons is not a new one. It is as ancient as time. However, in our society, we have become so technologically oriented that we often forget how to see magic in our everyday lives. We have forgotten how to "hear the corn singing." If we cannot quantify an experience, it does not exist. We rely on statistics to shape our minds into fearful alert patterns of diseases we are "likely" to get.*

In medicine there are specialists for every part of the body but few who know how, or who can take the time, to treat the body as a whole. HMOs are dominating the healthcare market, crippling wonderful physicians who want to give a "healing-care" to their patients rather than simply providing "Band-Aid care" as they are often forced to do. Although technology and the discoveries of medicine along with the spiritual teachings of physicians such as Deepak Chopra,[3] Larry Dossey,[4] Carl Hammerschlag,[5,6] Christiane Northrup,[7] Rachel Naomi Remen,[8] Bernie Siegel,[9,10] and Andrew Weil[11] have helped in our quest for a healthier society, rates of abuse, addiction, and violence continue to soar. Children killing children is commonplace. We have become a society that values the bottom line *more than the* life line. *Many of us often feel "dis-membered"— disconnected from life's magic. We need to be "re-membered" and reconnected to an essence of heart and spirit in order to heal from life's emotional and physical traumas.*

The stories and steppingstones in this part of the book will show you how to see and embrace nature as a natural world library *. . . in which a tree, a leaf, a feather, a butterfly, or even such annoying insects as flies can be used in much the same way as one uses a book to study important life lessons or to find comfort and healing during difficult times . . . and as the old man in the story tells us, "It takes a lot of practice. You can't be in a hurry."*

CHAPTER FOUR

Web of Relationships

"All the wilderness seems to be full of tricks
to drive and draw us up into God's light."

— John Muir[12]

A few weeks after Hurricane Iniki blew through our Island, some special friends from the neighborhood came by to help us clear our yard. There were many fallen trees, large lava-rock boulders, scraps of our roof as well as of the roofs of others, surfboards, and debris scattered everywhere. Mosquitoes and flies buzzed and whirred over the dead fish, which had washed onto our property from the ocean just a few hundred feet away, along with mounds of sand that had formed into dunes. It was especially painful to look at the beautiful trees and plants overturned, uprooted, lying helplessly on the earth. The powerful winds had turned a serene setting into a landscape of disaster.

After hours of backbreaking work loading and hauling the debris, making five trips to the dump with two huge canefield dump trucks and one front loader, we all took a rest. One of the men, Ray, came over to where I was standing.

"See that tree over there," Ray said as he pointed to a very large tree lying on its side in our front yard. Its roots were completely torn out of the ground and all of its once-green leaves had turned a dried-up brown color. The whole tree looked like it was dying or already dead. Ray continued very matter-of-factly. "That tree is a special tree on Kaua'i. It's called a 'Milo' tree and it's an endangered species. We're going to stand that tree up for you with the front loader and replant it."

With a somewhat disbelieving tone in my voice, I asked, "Are you sure you want to do that? You guys have done enough already—and, besides, the tree looks dead."

Ray laughed and said, "Oh, no, it'll be fine. We'll stand it back up and replant the roots in the ground. It'll grow back. You see, when a tree like that is knocked down and you stand it back up, it becomes even stronger than before, because its roots have to reach way down, deeper into the earth, to get its nourishment. Don't worry, Joyce, it'll grow back, just like I'm telling you."

Carefully, one of the front-loader trucks lifted the fallen tree until it was upright once again. As I watched, I felt a tangible shift within my body, as if I, too, were being "uprighted" after having been knocked over by the challenges of the move and my readjustment to a new lifestyle. I realized that perhaps the roots of my experience would have to reach down deeper into the soil of my new environment to get the spiritual nourishment I needed, so, like the tree, I could grow stronger than before. A smile came to my face as I realized that Ray had given me a gift of personal healing through the wisdom of nature.

About two months later I noticed bright-green leaves proudly sprouting forth from their once broken and dried branches. Ray was right . . . the Milo tree *is* stronger-looking, and its arm-like branches extend outward, as if embracing its new life.

Steppingstone Four

"In every seed is the promise of thousands of forests."

— Deepak Chopra[13, 14]

$\mathcal{S}$o many times in life we have experiences that leave us feeling knocked over and uprooted just like the Milo tree. Yet somehow, with the help of others, we are able to have our lives "uprighted" and "rerooted" once again. Usually we remember big kindnesses at the time they are happening, but too often their importance fades in the day-to-day "busyness" and demands of life. And in that busyness we may also forget to notice small blessings. Two such blessings come to mind right now.

In 1997 my sweet mother, Rose, died unexpectedly. While sitting at her bedside just an hour after her passing, my grief was so enormous I could barely breathe. Through my tears I noticed that the nurse who was telling me about the last moments of my mother's life was gently stroking her small, blanketed feet as if she were still alive. I felt as if my mother's spirit was being caressed by an angel. I am sure it was.

A second blessing occurred a few days later when I was flying back to Hawai'i. A young United Airlines flight attendant noticed I was dabbing tears from my eyes and tenderly asked if he could help. I told him about my mother's passing and we both had a lovely conversation about our mothers and how much they meant to us. Just before we landed, he came over and handed me a yellow origami lilly which he had just fashioned from a scrap of paper he found onboard. He said that it wasn't very much, but when I look at it maybe it would bring me comfort. The flower still sits on a shelf near a picture of my mother and me. As I look at this lilly, I am reminded to save the small kindnesses that touch my life daily, and enjoy the *spiritual interest* that accumulates as they continue to appreciate in value.

Although we are taught to save for the future, to start an investment retirement fund, so that we will be financially secure as we get older, I think it is just as important to start a "Blessing Fund," a place where we can deposit the day-to-day blessings, so that we may be spiritually secure as we go through life. Many of my clients who have had to go through chemotherapy have made "blessing boxes." They put in cards, notes, pictures, and momentos sent to them by loving people in their lives. Of course, you don't have to wait until you become ill to start a Blessing Fund. You can begin at any time.

Take a few moments and think about a blessing that happened to you today. A blessing can be a call from a close friend, a smile from your child, or the coffee someone in your office brought for you. It can be the warm greeting you received from the person behind the checkout stand at your local market or simply the ability to open your eyes and breathe in the blessing of life for another day. Write it down on an index card and place it in a special box, or write it in a blank book you can call your "Blessing Book." Like a safety deposit box where you keep your valuables, or a bankbook in which your deposits are recorded, you can withdraw a blessing whenever you feel spiritually in need.

CHAPTER FIVE

Winged Teachers

*". . . . It is only with the heart that one can see rightly;
what is essential is invisible to the eye."*

—Antoine de Saint-Exupery[15]

In our quest for a reconnection to the *heart-magic* within our lives, we often overlook the very place we must begin the search. The web of relationship with ourselves . . . with our own bodies. Nothing brought this home more clearly to me than through a teaching I received while attending a workshop on healing and guided imagery. Heart specialist and author Dr. Dean Ornish[16] asked our group what seemed like a strange question: "To which organ does the heart pump blood *first?*" Each of us answered, citing various organs and body parts, including the brain. Dr. Ornish told us that this question also stumped most medical students. The answer is, *the heart itself.* The heart must pump blood to itself before it can pump blood to any other organ. I thought this was a wonderful teaching, not only in relation to physiology. It is not the cognitive desires of the head that lead to heart fulfillment; we must first take care of the needs of the heart—our *heartsongs*—in order to feel fulfilled.

How many of us remember to listen to our heartsongs, to follow their melodies, even in the face of opposition? So often we find that the channels to our dreams are clogged, preventing us from connecting with our "bliss station," to use mythologist Joseph Campbell's term. When we disconnect from life's magic, in a sense we experience a spiritual heart attack. The veins and arteries that carry our soul's nourishment become blocked by the "shoulds" and "have-to's" of daily life . . . by what I call the "cholesterol of the soul."

So how do we stay connected to our heartsongs in the face of distractions, obstacles, and oppositions? In relation to this question, a story comes to mind of a teaching I received unexpectedly while watching a young man from the Dine' (Navajo) tribe tie a sacred water drum.

Wendall was going to use this drum for our evening gathering at his family's home. The uniqueness of this particular drum is that it is tied and untied with each use. Its base is a small black kettle, which is filled about a third of the way with water. A round piece of hide is soaked and stretched across the top of the drum and then tied by placing a small round stone under the hide—like a knob—and tying it securely with a rope. The rope is wrapped around each stone until seven are used. Once tied, the sound of the drum is not easily forgotten. Its beat is rapid in order to accompany special prayer chants.*

There are many stories connected with this particular drum, but my favorite was told to me by a Navajo spiritual leader I respectfully call Uncle. The story goes that one day a group of brothers went out hunting for food. They were gone for a very long time and their sister became worried about them. When she went out to look for them, she found them dead. They were sitting upright on the field, each holding his shield, waiting to say good-bye to their sister before they went to the spirit world.

She immediately returned to the village, fetched the kettle she used to cook for them, and filled it with water. She brought the water-filled kettle to the battlefield, took the hide from her brothers' shields, and placed it over the kettle. Taking the rope that fastened the hide to the hoop of the shield, she tied the hide to the kettle. Having completed her task, she gave the kettle to her brothers, saying, "Now you can go to the spirit world and always be close to the heart-beat of your sister."

Now, as I watched Wendall tie the drum, I noticed several flies land on his arms. Soon more flies landed on his hands, face, legs, and even on the moist deerskin hide. Kneeling on the rough, pebbled earth, securing the softened deer hide tightly stretched over the drum kettle between his knees and thighs, Wendall tried to swat them away by shrugging his shoulders, without letting go of the tension with which he held the drum . . . but to no avail. The buzzing flies stayed.

I thought to myself, "Why not just get up and move? Ugh, the flies are so annoying and distracting. They can ruin even the best of occasions." But Wendall stayed with the drum. His attention remained

---

*Although the custom of each tribe may vary, this drum is usually considered a male instrument and is not used by women. There are exceptions occasionally.

fixed on what he was doing, until the drum was fully tied. He then picked up his drumstick and drummed a few prayer chants into it, a way of tuning it up.

After he finished singing, I went up to him and asked, "Why didn't you just move to another spot and try to get rid of the flies? They seemed to be so distracting, yet you ignored them and continued on. I probably would have just moved."

Wendall laughed and said, "Well, Sister, it's like this. This drum is the heartbeat . . . and those little flies, well, they are our relatives, too. They are here to teach us something. You see, in life there are always distractions . . . things that annoy us, just when we are doing something that is really important to us. There are always flies. But my uncle taught me that when you begin to tie a drum like this, you stay with it . . . nothing is to get in the way . . . and whatever does come up is there to help you focus even more. Stay connected to your heartbeat and you'll be okay."

To this day, whenever flies come around me, I cannot help but smile and inwardly acknowledge these little creatures of nature as both "relative" and "teacher" and silently I say, "Thank you."

Steppingstone Five

HEARTSONG MEDITATION

*"It is in the interludes between being in company
that we talk to ourselves."*

—Maya Angelou[17]

As I read the above quote in the ending paragraph of Maya Angelou's inspirational book, *Even the Stars Look Lonesome*, I could not help but think of Wendall's teaching about the drum and the importance of staying connected to our heartsongs.

I am aware that in our busy and often noisy world the need for silence and quietude becomes as essential as the air that we need to breathe. This steppingstone is designed to help you find that solitude and honor the silence. By honoring the silence, perhaps as Ms. Angelou says, "....in the quietude we may even hear the voice of God."

- Begin by sitting in a comfortable position. Close your eyes and take a few slow, deep breaths, gently inhaling through your nose and exhaling through your mouth.

- Next ask yourself "What do I need (or need to know) most in my life right now?"

- When you have your answer, place your hand over your heart and remain very still, continuing to breathe comfortably.

- Remembering that your heart is your personal drum, become aware of its beat . . . its rhthym. Remain in that position for as long as your time will permit. For example, if you are at work, perhaps you only have a ten-minute break or a lunch hour. At home, you may have more time in the evening. Be respectful of whatever time you have at the moment.

- Next become aware of the message that your "heart-drum" is giving to you. This message is your *heartsong*. Perhaps take a moment to write it down on a notepad or in a journal. One woman with whom I worked told me that she wrote her heart-song message on an index card and she carries it with her like an affirmation card.

- Remember there are always "flies" that may try to distract your attention. Notice what these annoyances are in your life that distract your attention from something that is important to you . . . your heartsong. Once you become aware of those distractions, write them down and become familiar with them. Like the flies, when these distractions cross your path, they can become your "winged teachers" reminding you to once again reconnect to your heartsong.

- Close this meditation by returning to the beginning position, close your eyes, place your hand over your heart, take a few slow, deep breaths, and in your personal quietude smile and say, "Thank you."

CHAPTER SIX

Butterfly Magic

"From cocoon forth a butterfly
As lady from her door
Emerged , a summer afternoon,
Repairing everywhere. . . .

—Emily Dickinson[18]

nother relative of nature I think of as a winged teacher is the butterfly. Universally viewed as a symbol of transformation and healing, butterflies entrance, delight, and embrace the hearts of those who seek an understanding of personal growth and change. A story comes to mind here as told to me by Terry Tafoya, a psychologist and traditional Storyteller from the Warm Springs Tribe. I share it with you in the way that I remember it.

. . . . And so it is said a long, long time ago there were two Caterpillar People who were very much in love. One day a sad thing happened and the Caterpillar Man died. The heart of the Caterpillar Woman was broken. She didn't want to see anyone or talk to anyone and so she wrapped her sorrow around her like a shawl. Then she began walking and walking . . . and while she walked, she cried.

Caterpillar Woman walked for a whole year, and because the earth is a circle, she returned to the very place from which she had begun walking. The Creator took great pity on her, saying, "You have suffered too long. Now it is the time to step into a new world of color . . . a new world of great beauty." Then the Creator clapped hands twice . . . and the Woman burst forth from the shawl as a beautiful butterfly. And it is told that this is why the butterfly is a symbol of renewal for many communities . . . it tells us that at the end of all suffering, there is the gift of relief.

Spiritually, this ancient story provides us with an important teaching about healing and renewal. Scientifically, there is also another story which can help us to see how each stage of the butterfly's transformation parallels our own.

One spring day back in 1987, a very dear friend of mine, Diana Linden, a neurophysiological biologist at Occidental College, and I were discussing the use of metaphors to explain science. Diana enjoyed using stories to teach biology to her classes and I enjoyed listening to Diana talk about her amazing research into muscular dystrophy. During this visit, Diana asked me how I viewed healing. Pondering my response for a moment, an image of a butterfly came to mind. "When I think of healing, I think about the butterfly. You know, we are like a caterpillar crawling around, until at one point or another, we go inside our cocoon and transform into a butterfly." Chuckling a bit, Diana said, "Oh, Joyce, that's not exactly what happens. You're leaving out a big part of the process of transformation." She went on to tell me the story.

> *As most of us know, there are four stages to the butterfly's transformation . . . the Egg, the Caterpillar, the Chrysalis, and the Emerging Butterfly. What most of us don't know is what makes the metamorphosis possible . . . what changes the caterpillar into a butterfly. This is the part you are reeally going to like. Caterpillars have special cells in their bodies called "imaginal discs," which contain all the seeds of change."*

Imaginal discs, I echoed within myself. Diana was right, I loved it! As a matter of fact, even though I really didn't know what they were, I wanted to run right out and buy some imaginal discs for myself. I knew that I could certainly use something magical to help me release my personal seeds of change whenever I felt stuck in one place or another in my life. "Where can I get some?" I humorously quipped. Diana laughed along with me and then continued.

> *You see, the caterpillar prepares for this great change by eating and eating. When it is big enough, it shakes its body and sheds its skin, which it has now outgrown . . . shakes and sheds, shakes and sheds. Then just at the right time, it finds a leaf or a branch and attaches itself by weaving a thin silkened thread and a small pad, becoming what is known as* the chrysalis. *The chrysalis is a hardened skin that develops and protects the caterpillar as it goes through its changes. Inside of the chrysalis the caterpillar completely breaks down in structure, becoming a soupy-like substance.*

Diana went on to explain that it was only at the point of this breakdown that the imaginal discs release the seeds of change contained within, allowing the caterpillar to transform itself into a beautiful butterfly . . . as the magic of metamorphosis completes itself.

After hearing Diana's description of this amazing process of biological change, I felt especially stirred, because I was preparing to teach a new workshop at an upcoming psychotherapy conference on the use of metaphor in transformational healing. Until this moment I had been unable to generate any new ideas for this workshop. I felt stuck and frustrated. But now, savoring the concept of *imaginal discs*, as the source of metamorphosis for the butterfly, I could begin to envision a model of healing that was rooted in nature and powerfully relevant for people.

With great enthusiasm I rushed out to The Nature Company, a local store, and bought many books on the metamorphosis of the butterfly in hopes of finding a way to translate this scientific information into tangible teachings. I found what I was looking for in a book entitled *Butterfly & Moth*[19] by Paul Whalley, which beautifully illustrated and described each of the stages and combined it with the knowledge Diana shared with me. As this model of transformational healing and change began to unfold, I realized that so often in life we all go through the greatest times of fear, uncertainty, darkness, feeling like "I can't take one more thing." Then somehow, after what could be called a "moment of miracle," we find the inner strength . . . our own imaginal discs . . . to go on and eventually experience a breakthrough in our personal and spiritual growth.

And so it is with the greatest awe and respect for this graceful relative of nature . . . this winged teacher of change . . . that I share the following stories and steppingstones as they relate to each stage of the butterfly—and to our human ability to embrace and achieve the magic of change.

Steppingstone Six

"It's what you are meant to become. It flies with beautiful wings and joins the earth to heaven. It drinks only nectar from flowers and carries the seeds of love from one flower to another."

—Trina Paulus[20]

Journey with me as we take a closer look at how each of the four stages of the butterfly parallels the passages we experience in our quest for personal growth, change, and healing. After you have read each passage, write or draw your thoughts as they relate to that particular passage.

The First Passage:
New Beginnings

In the world of the butterfly, I learned that after a time of an elaborate courtship dance with the sole or "soul" purpose of attracting the opposite sex and mating, the female selects just the right plant on which to lay her eggs. She does this so that her eggs have a safe home on which to hatch. Paralleling this first stage we find the importance of creating a safe environment in which all new ideas, relationships, and personal awarenesses have the opportunity of developing. Without this safe environment, nothing positive develops. We need support and encouragement to go on.

I remember a time when I was in the fourth grade and was given an assignment to make a map of the world. Loving art, I did this assignment with great enthusiasm. However, I did not have blue paint to use for the water. I only had red paint and I didn't have the money to go out and buy blue paint. I worked for hours detailing the map in the best way that I knew how and proudly brought it into my classroom. We were each asked to show our work and when I stood before the class, holding the large poster-size map I had painted, the teacher commented, "What is all that red? We all know that the water is blue." At that moment the class laughed and I began to shake with embarrassment. I never raised my hand to volunteer for anything in that class again. My teacher's classroom was not a safe "leaf" for my "eggs" of childhood creativity.

As I look back on that experience today, I can see its positive influence on my life. I know that when I teach a workshop or see a new client, the most important thing for me to focus upon is creating a supportive environment so that each person can feel safe exploring and discovering new ideas and choices.

Personal Reflections: New Beginnings

Think back to the moment when you had a new idea that you were so excited about and went to share it with someone.

How did that person respond?

What was he or she doing when you were talking?

Was he looking around or was she glancing at her watch at the time?

Did you get the message to go on, or forget it?

Take stock. If someone new is coming into your business, how do you welcome him or her? Was there a note, flowers, an invitation to lunch . . . or was the person just shown to his or her office and told, "If you need something, call?" Is your environment—whether it be home, classroom, or business—one that nurtures an inner well-spring of creative passion? In order to encourage positive change, healing, and empowerment, it is essential to provide a supportive "leaf" on which people feel safe to lay the eggs of their ideas. This stage protects and incubates that which is new.

The Second Passage:
The Caterpillar: You Gotta Crawl Before You Fly

Have you ever said to yourself any of the following statements? "I am not happy in this relationship, I am outgrowing my partner, job, or lifestyle." "I know that I need to make some changes in my life." "I need to shed my skin and become a new person." "I'm not happy living in this body." Well, if you have pondered any of these thoughts, it is a good indicator that you have entered the second passage of *Breakthrough.*

Like the caterpillar, we know it is time for a change in our lives. We may express feelings of being bored with life, of wanting to move on in some way. Sometimes people may gain a great deal of weight during this stage, saying they feel like eating everything in sight. I certainly did this prior to my move to Kaua'i, which continued until recently, leaving me with a weight gain of almost fifty pounds. I remember a good friend of mine in Los Angeles telling me that in Yoga teachings they say that just before a great change in life, one gains a great deal of weight. Then when the change completes itself, the weight seems to fall away. I welcomed this bit of news with gleeful anticipation.

Oftentimes, there just seems to be an overall sense of discontentment with life, as it is in this second passage, but discontentment is not necessarily negative. It is can be used as a positive indicator pointing to the need for change in our lives or letting us know that change is on the way whether we have asked for it or not. This is particularly true of adolescents. They don't like their bodies, hair, or selves in general. It is as if teenagers are in a psychic search for another form; however, they don't seem to know what that form is as yet.

How well I remember those feelings vividly. I remember looking at my small breasts, wondering if they would ever grow . . . would I ever wear a bra bigger than a 28-triple-A size? I knew that my body was changing, but I had no idea into what. I used to read all of the teen books at the time and bought over-the-counter creams which claimed miracle breast development. I would walk with my shoulders slouched in hopes nobody would notice that I only had bumps on my chest, or I would stuff my friend's bra (which was two sizes larger than mine) with cotton so that I appeared voluptuous overnight. I would lie in bed at night and pray that God would perform a miracle and bring me breasts by morning.

How can teenagers know consciously that they have the ability to become "butterflies," when they are still in their caterpillar-selves? Now that I am beginning menopause, I feel the inner stirrings of change once again. I do not really know where these changes in my feminine cycles will take me . . . how my dreams will change . . . what shape my body will take . . . in what new directions my work will lead me. I only know that my inner "itchings," as I like to think of them, are indicators to me that I am in my caterpillar stage.

Preparing for Change

Just how do we know when it is time to change? "You watch the sail, and feel the wind, and you just know inside when it is time to change." These are the words that were shared with me by a young man whose innate ability to sail the challenging oceans of Kaua'i matched the grace and vision possessed by the soaring eagles of the skies. On January 1, 1988, Leonard and I set out for an afternoon sail on his two-person catamaran. At one point I glanced up and noticed that his deeply set brown eyes were focused upwards towards the mast, while he skillfully maneuvered the sails with his long sun-browned fingers and manipulated the rudder with the toes of his bare foot. We were heavily tilted on our bow while the powerful winds carried us across the azure blue ocean with swift grace.

At another time the waves were increasing their height and intensity. Leonard motioned for me to change positions and move to the other side of the catamaran. After carefully wobbling my body across the small catamaran and steadying my balance, I asked the question I mentioned at the beginning of this section, "How do you know when it is time to change?" I thought that I was referring to the situation on the catamaran, but as I thought about it later, I realized that my question was far more about life in general than about an ocean adventure.

Perhaps this would be a good time to stop reading and ask yourself, "How do I know *when* it is time to change? What are my personal signals?" Use the following page to reflect upon these questions.

How Do I Know *When* It Is Time to Change? What are My Personal Signals?

Imaginal Discs . . . Seeds of Change

At this point you may be asking, "So what's the magic that's going to transform me from a caterpillar to a butterfly?" The answer is imaginal discs. Yes, like the butterfly each of us also has imaginal discs that contain all "seeds of change." These imaginal discs are our inner resources, interests, skills, and past learnings—just lying dormant and, in a sense, just waiting to be awakened . . . to be released. Just as the little caterpillar carries these cells within its fuzzy body, we too carry these cells within our caterpillar-stage selves . . . not knowing, consciously, that we even have them or what they can do for us when their "time" comes. I like to think of imaginal discs as our "winged assets" of change, enabling us to renew a sense of hope, recognizing that unseen possibilities are truly present to help us move forward, no matter what challenge or obstacle is placed in our paths.

As I write this, I think about an interview with Christopher Reeve I saw on the television news-magazine show, *20/20.* There he sat, strapped into his wheelchair, completely paralyzed as a result of a catastrophic fall from his horse, relying on a respirator for his very breathing. Yet while he and his wife acknowledged what had been taken from them because of the accident, the focus of their talk revolved around what they had together . . . love, belief, determination, faith, hope . . . their own imaginal discs to help transcend the physical limitations into a realm of spiritual achievement.

When we look at a little caterpillar, do we ever see these magical cells? No, not consciously. But they *are* there. These cells of change contain and protect all of the mystery that transforms the caterpillar into the butterfly.

Two stories come to mind here illustrating how the imaginal discs of two teenage boys were used to help each of them overcome personal limitations. Perhaps after you read these stories, you can take a moment to reflect upon your own hobbies, interests, and talents . . . your own "winged assets of change."

Skiing Algebra

There was a time some years ago when my youngest son, Casey, was in high school and failing good old algebra. A good friend of ours, Tom, was a math wizard and he generously volunteered to tutor Casey through his difficulties. No matter how hard Casey tried, he would get very anxious before a test and then fail. Tom knew that Casey knew the work, but as for many of us, his doubts about himself got in the way and blocked his potential growth, achievement, and confidence.

Knowing that Casey had the ability to pass but was stuck in his limited belief systems about his abilities to ever pass, I decided to try to awaken his Imaginal Discs. Casey is a wonderful skier. He loves every aspect of the sport and is confident in his abilities as a skier. Knowing this full well, I went into the den where Casey had been intensely pondering his upcoming test and said, "Casey, you really like skiing don't you?" Giving me his "Mom, what-are-you-up-to" look, he answered, "Of course . . . you know that I love it." I continued. "Casey, what do you like about it?" Now, I could guess what he liked about it, but that was not the point. *My* knowing has nothing to do with *his* knowing. He went on to tell me in great detail what he liked about it, still looking at me skeptically.

I continued. "Tell me, what happens when you decide to go on a more advanced slope, or on one that you have never skied before?" Casey answered me almost immediately without a pause. "Challenged," was his response. I repeated the word slowly, "Challenged." I continued, "How do you feel when you are just ready to get off that ski-lift and you really don't know what is up ahead?" I was also using my hand to demonstrate the upward climb of the lift. Again Casey's response was quick and forward. "Challenged, excited to get off the lift and ski the slopes." Then somewhat annoyed he said, "Mom, where are you going with all this skiing stuff?" But rather than answer at this point, I persisted a bit more. "Casey, what about the moguls (those are little hills in the mountains that bounce and bump the skier as he or she skis down the slopes) or the trees, rocks, or other things that come up as you ski. Do they bother you?"

Once again, with a humorous, yet somewhat annoyed tone, Casey answered, "No Mom, they just make it more fun." Finally, I stopped my questioning and simply looked directly in his eyes and with a soft, clear voice I said, "Casey, then *SKI ALGEBRA . . . SKI ALGEBRA.*" Casey smiled and was silent. I smiled back and said, "See ya' later" and walked out of the room. About a week later, Casey called me at work and with great excitement in his voice said, "Guess what! I got a 97 on my test. Mom, I SKIED ALGEBRA."

Casey has since graduated from college and works with children who have serious emotional challenges to overcome in their lives. He tells me that to this day, whenever he faces a difficult decision or an obstacle in his life, he tells himself to "*ski*" it . . . and while remembering this, he laughs.

Keys

On a visit to a residential treatment center in Oregon, I had the opportunity of working in one of the cottages, which housed twenty-four children who were described as having the most serious problems in the school. I decided to work with these children, ranging in age from eight years old to seventeen years old, in a large group. The staff wondered how this would work since many of the children were identified as being violent, delusional, dissociated from reality, and unable to sit still for a long period of time. I wondered as well, since I had never worked with such a group before.

I noticed a large round hand-held drum hanging on the wall as I entered the cottage and asked if we could use it. "Sure" was the enthusiastic response of the cottage manager. My thought was to first tell the children about the drum and how it is a connection to their heartbeat. Since most of these children are so disconnected from their own heartsongs, I felt this would be a good way to reintroduce them to their own rhythms. My second intention was to pass the drum in the circle and have each of the children hit it once with the drumstick, thereby putting their "voice" into it.

I then went into the gymnasium and asked the children and staff to sit on the hard wood floor to form a large circle. I began to spread out many of the things I had brought, such as sweetgrass, sage, a shell, feathers, my grandmother's shawl, salt from Hawai'i, and my two endearing turtle puppets, B.T. (Big Turtle) and L.T. (Little Turtle) . . . my medicine. I explained that in many cultures medicine is not something that just comes in bottles; instead medicine can be found in all aspects of life, such as in stories, rocks, plants, and many things of nature, as well as in those special objects given to us by special people.

A young boy sitting next to me proudly told me that he had a drum, some feathers, and a medicine bag his grandfather, a respected Lakota tribal elder, had given to him some years ago. I leaned over and whispered, "Well, what are you waiting for, go and get your special things." He was clearly delighted and went to his room, accompanied by a staff member, and came back in a few moments with his very sacred treasures . . . his medicine.

I continued to lay out the special things I had brought to share with the group. Somehow the veil of mental and emotional illness that seemed to separate us slowly began to lift and I was simply sitting in a circle of children. As I began to talk about how we each have special things that make us feel good, the boy sitting to my left began to talk rapidly and told me he wanted to share something that was important to him with the group, too. It was his "medicine." I excused him also and he went to his room to get his special gift. When he came back he had many pieces of paper on which "keys" were drawn. All kinds of keys. Car keys, door keys, storage-box keys, and pictures of keys he had drawn on multiple pieces of paper. In a rapid-fire fashion, he began telling me all about his keys.

As he talked, it became apparent that the other children in the group were becoming increasingly annoyed with his diatribe. One girl huffed and said, "We heard this before; that's all he ever talks about." I simply acknowledged her statement with a nod and turned to the boy and said, "You know, keys are so very important. Without keys I couldn't start my car, I couldn't open the door to my house, or for that matter, I wouldn't be able to lock it in order to keep everything safe inside. Yes, keys are *very* important."

This boy with the cinnamon-colored hair and smiling blue eyes quieted his chattering and moved closer to me. The other children in the group slightly nodded their heads in agreement. Yes, keys are very important. For this boy, they were his medicine . . . the keys to his inner life.

Since that time, I have returned to Oregon many times, and I have had special visits with Joey. I heard how the sensitive staff have continued to help Joey on a daily basis use his "obsession" with keys for unlocking the hidden pathways to his private world. Joey can now draw a picture of himself, a tree with apples on it, and even tell me a story. One story is about a little bird who found the key to his bird cage, so he can open the door any time he wants to and fly away. On my last trip, I learned that Joey no longer talks about keys, but is interested in cameras. He is busy taking pictures of life.

"Winged Assets of Change"

Use the following page to write down the things that you enjoy doing in your life, be they hobbies, interests, or things that are simply delightful to do, such as watching a sunset, the first snow of the season, birds singing, or your favorite flowers.

By identifying our own imaginal discs we are better equipped to confront our greatest struggles and fears with a certain confidence. This is the confidence that allows us to overcome self-doubt, fear, and pain so that we may reach a rich Soul life filled with joy and empowerment.

My Imaginal Discs

The Third Passage
The Chrysalis: Dark Spaces of Change

This third passage creates the greatest attention as to the mystery of change. With the chrysalis completely formed, the caterpillar is now ready to "break down" and have its special cells, the imaginal discs, release the seeds of change. While the chrysalis appears inactive, quiet on the outside, the most amazing and dramatic changes take place on the inside. *It is during this stage that the magic of transformation takes place.* Like the butterfly, it is in this stage that our greatest change occurs as well.

Our chrysalis stage is often marked as a peak time of "not know-ing." It is a period of withdrawal, not wanting to socialize, often wanting to hide and not deal with the outside world, with a given struggle, or with a certain situation. I often hear clients say, "I just want to pull the covers over my head and not face anyone . . . I want to wake up and have this problem gone . . . I can't see a way out of this situation . . . my life feels hopeless." Life often feels dark and iso-lated with little space for outer movement. Although some people view these feelings as symptoms of depression or anxiety, I choose to view these same symptoms as indicators of being in this third stage . . . the chrysalis . . . the place where the greatest change can occur.

Like the caterpillar, which must break down into a soupy, gel-like substance before releasing its seeds of change, so too do we need to learn how to break down old limiting belief systems about ourselves in order to transform from our caterpillar-like selves into empowered human beings capable of reaching our full-winged potential.

How often do we try to hold on to our old caterpillar selves only to find that if we continue to do so, we never discover our fly-away-butterfly selves? Think of all the survivors' groups with more coming into existence every day. As an alternative, I dream about *thriver* groups. Although surviving is an important stage in the quest for healing from trauma, it is not the *only* stage. Thriving is the next stage. It is the *butterfly-taking-flight* stage. In *Women Who Run With the Wolves*, Clarissa Pinkola Estes writes, "If we only stay as survivors without moving to thriving, we limit ourselves and cut our energy to ourselves and our power in the world to less than half." In other words, we stay caterpillars, we don't become butterflies. Remember: *Scars are markers of where we have been, not where we are going.*

The Navajo Rug

One afternoon I received a phone call from a distraught mother of a teenage girl I used to see in therapy. It seemed that her daughter Becky had a memory triggered and emotionally revealed a time when she was sexually molested by a former male neighbor who was a young adult at the time.

Becky came in with her mother and father to talk about this memory. Her mother revealed that she had also been abused as a child and that this situation was extremely difficult for her even though she had been in her own therapy and was doing very well. Becky's father was grateful to be included in this therapy as he, too, had many feelings of sadness and anger at what happened to his little girl.

Slumped in a corner of my couch, Becky's head was curled downward as she expressed herself. Looking at her, it was as if she were crawling within her own chrysalis so that she could feel a protection around her while she spoke. In between soft sobs, Becky said that she wondered if she could ever be whole again . . . if she could ever be clean again . . . is this why she was feeling the way she was feeling about herself, which was never good enough, never pretty enough.

As Becky was talking, an image of a sheep came into my mind, followed by an image of a wonderful old Navajo woman sitting by a great loom weaving a Navajo rug. Since we had worked together before, Becky knew that I used images and storytelling as the foundation of my therapy. After telling Becky about these images, I began to tell her what I had learned about Navajo weaving. "A weaver takes care of her own sheep. She shears the wool . . . she cleans the wool . . . then she spins and colors it, preparing it to become yarn. She then sits before her great loom and begins to weave from her visions . . . it is like a ceremony for her. She also sings the whole time she is weaving. As she sits there, a beautiful pattern begins to emerge. The pattern tells a story." I went on to say that I had learned that in the Navajo way, the weaver always weaves a mistake into each rug, to remind us that all things of beauty in life are not perfect.

"It might take a week, it might take a month, or it might take three months . . . it depends on how long the weaver wants to sit by that loom and work. . . . And everyone knows that a Navajo rug is one of the strongest rugs made. It lasts for centuries and is known for its beauty." Then I said, "You know, it is important to remember something . . . *THE SHEEP IS NOT THE RUG AND THE WOOL IS NOT THE RUG . . . IT IS ONLY PART OF THE RUG . . . IT IS UP TO THAT WEAVER TO TAKE THAT WOOL AND WEAVE IT INTO THE BEAUTIFUL, STRONG RUG IT BECOMES.*" I then remained silent.

Becky's sobbing stopped and a smile emerged on her face. Her mom and dad leaned closer to each other and held hands. I looked meaningfully at each one of them and repeated, "The sheep is not the rug . . . " And the session ended.

About four weeks later, Becky came bubbling into my office carrying a card and a gift for me. She sat close while I opened the gift. It was a replica of a woman in traditional Navajo dress, sitting by a loom with a half-woven Navajo rug on it. I then opened the card, which had a strong Native American warrior on the front. Inside Becky had written a note that still sits on my desk. She wrote, "I am not the Sheep . . . I AM THE RUG."

Up until this point, Becky was in her survivor-caterpillar stage of getting through life . . . doing the best she knew how. But she was clearly ready to move on . . . to begin to thrive . . . to transform from caterpillar to emerging butterfly.

Personal Reflections: Life's Gift Wrapping

Staying with quiet space and a time of not knowing—not having clear-cut answers or quick solutions to our problems—withdrawal from the outside world— is not often honored in our society. We are supposed to have the answers and be able to come up with solutions at the drop of a hat. Yet, nature tells us that this is a critical time in the life cycle of change. It is important to remember that all creatures of nature have a time of withdrawal, dormancy, or hibernation. There is a life-cycle pattern that allows for a time of cocooning. Think about the cycles of the seasons. There is Fall, when the leaves change from green to vibrant colors, only to become brittle and then fall off the trees. Followed by a coldness, a bareness . . . Winter. And through the cold there is an absence of color vibrancy . . . all is asleep. The season of Winter is most like this Chrysalis stage—all the changes are taking place on an inner level.

Likewise, beneath the chrysalis of the earth, within the womb of her caves, life is preparing to regenerate. This regeneration reveals itself during the next season, Spring. It is a reawakening of life, of nature. It is a time of emergence. Spring is playful, passionate, and fluttering. And then it slowly changes once again into Summer. There is often intense heat, a dramatic change from the seasons that came before . . . a time when the youthful growth of Spring turns into the mature passion of Summer. The four cycles of the butterfly are very much like the four seasons of nature. There must be the season of Chrysalis before the season of Emerging Butterfly.

Perhaps you feel frustrated with your personal growth or impatient with your ability to expand new ideas. Use the space provided on the following page to reflect upon what the chrysalis passage means to you; perhaps you will be able to see that this dark space of change is truly life's gift wrapping. Open the gift wrap. I hope you will discover a new *present* waiting.

What Cocooning Means to Me

The Fourth Passage
Emerging Butterfly: Wings Happen

A long time ago I heard a story about a man who found a large cocoon and decided to take it home to watch the butterfly inside emerge. As I remember it, the man watched and watched until one day he noticed a tiny opening in the cocoon. He thought the butterfly was struggling to make its way out of the cocoon and that something must be wrong. So he decided to help the butterfly along by making a larger slit for it to emerge with greater ease. When the butterfly finally came out, its wings were somewhat shriveled and small and its body misshapen. The man thought that the wings would spread out in a few hours, but they did not. Instead the butterfly was unable to fly . . . it was crippled for life. Although the man was well meaning, he did not know that there was a purpose for the struggle; it was nature's way of propelling the body's fluid into the wings of the butterfly so that it could emerge and ultimately fly with strength and beauty.

This story shows us that even though the butterfly is completely formed, it has to use all of its pulsating strength to push itself through its protective chrysalis into the light. It then hangs upside-down, gently fluttering its still-wet wings. You see, even though the butterfly is fully developed and born into the world, it is not quite ready for flight. If the wet-winged butterfly is rushed along, it will be crippled for life. The butterfly knows when it is time to fly . . . no one has to tell it or coax it.

In our own lives, the beginning of this fourth passage is often marked by our taking more and more risks . . . flexing our newly acquired wings, so to speak. On an inner level we experience the first inklings of hopefulness after a dark time of unconscious change. This passage is a time of awakenings . . . of "ah-ha" insights . . . of breaking through our cocoon. It is critical to our well-being that we not be pushed during this stage but supported to move forward at our own pace. Just as the butterfly awaits the right time to fly, at a certain point we will feel ready to assert ourselves in the world.

We begin to feel more secure with our new learnings and abilities. We may take that leap of faith to change jobs, enroll in a class we have thought about for some time, initiate a new friendship or relationship, or take that long-envisioned trip. Whatever outer action is chosen, we are ready to fly with new wings of vision and courage.

Recognizing My Wings

How do we know when we are in this fourth passage? Review the following sentences and see if they sound familiar. "I feel like I'm finally beginning to see the light at the end of the tunnel." "I feel like I could soar." "I can finally hear the music in my life again." "These ideas are finally taking off." If you have experienced any of these feelings, you will know that you are well into the fourth passage of change.

Whether we are creatively involved in a project, exploring new relationships, or encountering life's challenges, we can see the four passages leading to the miracle of change in all that we do . . . if we just take the time to look. Sometimes we look, but do not see. We listen, but do not hear. We touch, but do not feel. For me the butterfly speaks the language of healing and determination. She flutters by and invites our attention to her silent magic . . . her ability to crawl, to withdraw, to break down, to reform, to *break through*, and to soar. We can soar.

CHAPTER SEVEN

Talking Leaves

*"Nature is but another name for health,
and the seasons are but different states of health."*

—Henry David Thoreau[21]

With drooping shoulders and a saddened, sunken expression, fifty-two-year-old Lynn was a woman who felt her life was over since entering menopause. She had started hormone replacement therapy some six months ago but still felt dead inside. Her doctor wanted to prescribe antidepressants, which Lynn did not want to take. No amount of explaining to her on an intellectual level about the hormonal changes taking place changed how she felt about herself. Lynn described her feelings as "dead and useless."

One autumn day during a hike through her favorite park, Lynn noticed the changes that were taking place around her. As she looked at the vibrant colors of the leaves, Lynn remembered something she had learned years before from one of her biology classes, namely that nothing in nature is really lost, it just transforms.

Lynn decided to continue her hike and find five leaves from different trees or bushes and then sit down with them and let them teach her something she needed to know. Lynn found herself laughing out loud and commented, "Oh, great—talking leaves!"

As is often the case, answers do not come at the drop of a hat. Sometimes personal discoveries appear in more ingenious ways than we could ever envision. Lynn's experience was no different. She found five leaves from trees along the way, but when she sat down with them, nothing happened. She turned them over, spread them on the ground, laid them on a nearby rock, but still nothing. They were silent.

Heading home, she thought to herself, "Oh well, this is stupid anyway . . . talking to leaves . . . hmmm, I better not tell anyone or they'll *reeealy* think I'm losing it."

Later that day, Lynn went out to her backyard and found herself looking at a tree that she had planned to cut down. For some time it hadn't been producing any new fruit and she had been advised that "because it didn't seem to have any life to it," it would be better to cut it down and replace it with a newer, fruit-bearing tree. Thinking back to her earlier time in the park and her talking leaves experience, Lynn felt compelled to pick five leaves from this particular tree and repeat her living metaphor exercise and let the leaves teach her something she needed to know. Looking very closely at each one, Lynn saw something she had not expected. She realized that the leaves still had a lot of life left in them. She had never looked at them closely before and had only taken the word of her gardener about how useless the tree had become.

It was at this moment that Lynn synthesized the experience into her own teaching. It was one of those "ah-ha" moments for her. Excitedly she quipped, "*I'm* like the leaves . . . like the tree. I have plenty of life in me, even though I'm changing. Nothing's going to cut me down, that's for sure."

From that time on whenever Lynn doubted her value during her changing-woman season, all she needed to do was talk to the leaves and the trees, because like very wise grandparents, they knew a lot about *relief*—about *re-leafing!*

Steppingstone Seven

LISTENING TO NATURE

"As the water reappeared,
so there reappeared willows, rushes, meadows,
gardens, flowers, and a certain purpose in being alive."

—Jean Giono[22]

*P*erhaps like Lynn, you too are experiencing a time of changing seasons within your own life. Maybe you are questioning your purpose or value . . . feeling lost, without a clear direction. Take a walk out into nature and pick up a rock, leaf, flower, or any other object that spiritually speaks to you or sparks your attention. Next hold that nature-object in your hands, close your eyes and ask it to teach you something important that can be of help to you right now. Pay attention to the ideas, images, or sensations that come to you. Each image, idea, or sensation becomes the messenger carrying a message of great importance. For Lynn, the leaves from the tree reminded her about the vibrancy that still existed within her own life.

What would those leaves say to you if you held them in your own hands? Feel free to use the remaining space on this page to jot down any thoughts or feelings that may come into your mind after this experience.

The One That Got
Away . . . Or Did It?

*"If one is lucky, a solitary fantasy can totally
transform one million realities."*

—Maya Angelou[23]

he lake was calm as we sat fishing off the side of a small
motorboat. It was the summer of 1979 when we went for a
family vacation in Lake Isabella, a small town a few hundred miles northeast of Los Angeles. My son Casey was determined to
catch his first fish. We stopped at the local fishing supply store and
stocked up on all the equipment we needed for our afternoon's outing:

bait, tackle, fishing pole, and so on. Hours passed as Casey patiently waited for something to tug at his line. Suddenly his pole began to bend and his big brown eyes filled with excitement. "Mom, Dad," he shouted, "I think I got something." We all watched as Casey held his pole steady and reeled in his fish. What looked like a pretty-good-sized fish slowly began to swish and swirl its way to the surface. Then our excitement quickly turned to disappointment. Rather than the expected catfish, there was a big, brown stick hanging at the end of Casey's pole. Eddie and I told him that he had done a great job and to keep on fishin'. Being the kind of determined kid that he was, Casey did just that. He continued to wait patiently for a fish. By the late afternoon, we agreed to give it up and head back to the dock.

As we tied our boat's line to the dock, we noticed other fishermen showing off their day's catch. We recognized one of the men because he had been fishing near us. He was holding up a full line with about ten large catfish hanging off of it. I guess he recognized us, too, and came over to see how Casey did. We told him that we didn't catch anything but had fun anyway. Casey quickly piped up and said, "Wait a minute, we did too catch something, *I* caught a stick!" And there he stood, proudly holding up the "fish stick" he had caught. The man was very kind and obviously knew how to talk to children, because he said, "Well son, you sure did catch somethin', and that's a mighty fine stick at that." Casey was beaming, knowing his day was a success.

It has been about twenty years since that afternoon and I still reflect on the important teaching Casey gave to me. As adults we often base our success on the bottom *line*, the finished product. Casey taught me that it is not the finished product that is as important as much as the ability to see past concrete reality and measure success with the full vision of our heart.

94

Steppingstone Eight

*"There is a purpose for our lives far grander and
more significant than perhaps we might ever have considered."*

—David McNally[24]

Keeping Casey's idea of personal success in mind, perhaps you have a fish-stick story of your own that you may have forgotten due to living in the fast track with all of its "accomplishments." The following ideas can help you reflect on what success really means to you, and maybe you'll be surprised at your delightful "catch" at the end of the day.

- First get a notepad and write everything that comes to your mind on the *personal* meaning of success. You can begin with a simple phrase such as "Success means. . . . "
- Next draw a circle, divide it into fourths, and write the word

"Family" in one quarter, "Business" in another, "Self" in the third quarter, and the word "Spiritual" in the fourth quarter. You may also use the circle provided on the next page.

- After you have divided your circle, go back to your list and write key words within each quarter. For example, if you have written "Success means inner peace," would you write "inner peace" in the quarter marked Family, Business, Self, or Spiritual? You can write the same phrase or word in more than one place.

- As you look at your circle, notice the areas of your life in which you have achieved success. You may notice a number of success words or phrases listed in one area and fewer in another. This Circle of Success exercise can help you discover which areas of your life are rich and others which may need more attention.

Circle of Success

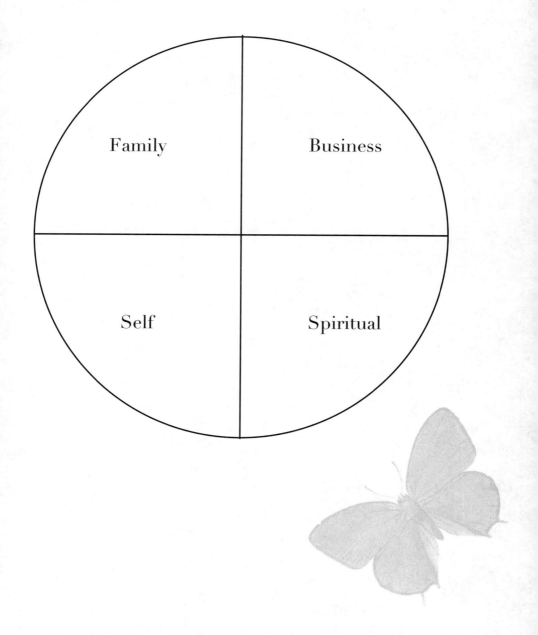

PART THREE

Restoring the Breath of Life

"The truth yields to nothing except growth:
it has no method which does not correspond to the
'method of the rose' - which is but to grow."

—Laurens van der Post[1]

Aloha is a Hawaiian word with many meanings. Among them are hello, spirit, and love, to name a few. I have also come to learn that there is another meaning, one that expands upon the concept that we are all connected by a web of relationship. During one of our classes, my friend and teacher, Kalani Flores, taught me that the root word "ha" in Aloha means breath. Not just breath as in the way we think of ordinary breathing, but breath that connects us to all of life . . . past, present, and future . . . both human and all species of plant and animal life from our natural world. Although there are other interpretations, Kalani went on to explain that the root word "Alo" means I greet you face to face. Therefore, by joining both of these root words together, the meaning of Aloha unfolds to say, "I greet you face to face with the breath of all of life."

Sometimes the challenges of undaunting trauma and pain threaten to choke the very breath of life right out of us. The thought of accomplishing a simple everyday task like making the bed, or getting dressed, becomes a major effort. We are continually being summoned by life's challenges to create new ways of meeting those challenges with a sense of dignity and hope. It is my hope that the stories shared in this part of the book will inspire you to face the obstacles that block your abilities to enjoy life, and restore a sense of inner balance and harmony . . . and the meaning of Aloha becomes infused with the very act of living.

CHAPTER NINE

Willie and the Taro Patch

"Nothing retains its own form; but Nature,
the greater renewer, ever makes up forms from forms.
Be sure there's nothing perishes in the whole universe;
it does but vary and renew its form."

—Ovid[2]

One day, some eight months after Hurricane Iniki, there was a knock on my door. A woman with whom I had worked in the shelter greeted me shyly. "I don't mean to bother you at home," Annie said, "but I need your help." I told her it was no bother at all and invited her into my home. (It's like that here in Kaua'i, your office is wherever you are at the moment.) With desperation in her voice, Annie asked if I would talk to her brother Willie. There had been a tragic accident several months earlier, in which Willie had accidentally shot and killed their brother, Daryl, while on a family hunting trip. On this day Daryl had not put on the brightly colored hunting vest they usually wore, and when he rustled through the bushes, Willie mistakenly thought the noise signaled a deer. Tragically it was not a deer but his younger brother. After the accident, Willie became severely depressed, angry, and was drinking too much. His violent outbursts provoked his wife to initiate legal action against him. He was put on probation with specific directions to join a substance abuse program and to learn to control his anger.

As a proud Hawaiian man, Willie is not comfortable talking about personal feelings in public, let alone to a group of strangers. Although he went to the substance-abuse groups initially, he found himself withdrawing and feeling more and more depressed. Willie's depression had deteriorated to such a point that he threatened to take a shotgun and kill himself. He now says that something he cannot explain stopped him from pulling the trigger. I told Annie that, of course, I would talk to him if he wanted to talk with me. She said she would bring him to my office and then leave us alone. It was clear how much she loved her brother.

Annie did as she promised. She brought Willie to my office, introduced us, and left us alone to *talk story*. As I closed the door, I wondered just how we would begin. With large, sun-browned forearms folded, Willie sat across from me in an old, slightly tattered rattan chair. Willie's gentleness was quite apparent, even through his broad Hawaiian frame. His true heartsongs seemed to be silenced by the intense pain he was living. At this point in his life, alcohol and anger were his only means of expressing a pain he could not tolerate.

Instinctively, I knew not to ask direct questions about the accident . . . it would be like picking at raw wounds. Instead I chose a softer, more indirect approach, one that is not only culturally respectful, but more comfortable for me. I began by sharing things about myself— not just about Joyce, the therapist, but more important about Joyce, the person. In telling Willie about myself, I shared stories of how I had learned to look at nature as containing all the medicine to help us heal from struggles. I was talking about spiritual medicine, not the medicine found in bottles. I talked about the hurricane and told the story of the Milo tree in my front yard and how nature has a way of talking to us and helping us in many ways. Willie must have liked what occurred in that first session, because he wanted to come back.

Over the course of many meetings, we never spoke directly about alcohol, violence, or his brother's death. Yet all of the issues were addressed within the ebb and flow of the stories we shared . . . and these stories seemed to act like a cushion on which Willie could rest his pained and weary soul.

One such story I shared with Willie early in our counseling was about a time I had participated in a sweat lodge ceremony in which I thought I was truly going to die. I explained to Willie that the sweat lodge is a Native American ceremony for purification and prayer.*

The lodge itself is a dome-shaped structure, made with a willow frame and covered with blankets (or other available material) so that it is very dark inside, symbolizing a womb. There is a round pit dug out in the center of the lodge, in which large lava rocks, which have been baked in an outside fire for hours, are brought in and placed in the pit, one by one. The lodge is low, so participants must crawl in as tiny children, and there is no room to stand. The people sit around the pit and wait for the leader to begin the prayers. I shared what I had learned about the sacredness of the rocks and how they are referred to as Grandfathers, Grandmothers, Rock People, or relatives,

---

*Each lodge and ceremony may differ, depending on the tribe and leader.

depending on the leader. They are not viewed as inanimate objects but as sacred members of a larger circle of creation.

I told Willie that in a sweat lodge there are four rounds . . . just as there are four seasons . . . four directions . . . and three trimesters of pregnancy with birth in the fourth. I told him how I wanted to run out during the second round because the heat was so intense. My heart was pounding louder and faster than the drums outside and I felt as if I could not breathe. But I learned that all I wanted to run away from was my own fear . . . my own pain. The sweat lodge leader sensed my fear and desperation through the darkness of the lodge and gently comforted me by telling me to put my face close to Mother Earth and "breathe into her . . . feel the coolness, let go of your fear . . . the earth will take care of you." I did as he suggested and was able to stay for all four rounds. I emerged from the ceremony with an inner strength I had never before experienced.

My intention through relating this story was to provide Willie with a sense of reassurance in the counseling process. I wanted him to know that I understood that there might be times he would want to run away from painful issues, and that facing his stuggles could literally feel life-threatening. But by staying and confronting his fears, he could emerge with a renewed sense of inner strength and well-being.

Within a few weeks of listening to stories about rocks, leaves, flies, butterflies, the ocean, and hurricanes, Willie slowly began to share stories of his family . . . of his experiences as a young boy growing up on Kaua'i, hunting, fishing, working in the taro fields. Willie's face would light up especially when he spoke about his children and his new grandson, whom he named Kahana, which means *turning point* in Hawaiian. It became clear how important it was for him to be the one to tell the stories to his children . . . and his grandson. He is the grandfather, the carrier of stories from one generation to the next.

During this time, I began taking Hawaiian lessons from Kalani

Flores. Kalani doesn't teach in a hurried fashion. He teaches the stories woven within the words. One night Kalani was teaching about numbers and began to talk about the number *four*. In Hawaiian four is *eha* (Āhá, with emphasis on the *ha*). He said that the root word is *ha* and in Hawaiian, *ha* means *breath of life*. He then drew a picture of the taro plant, which is still a staple food source for the Hawaiian people. He said that the stalk that connects the taro to the leaves is the *ha* . . . the breath of life. The taro plant itself at the base of the *ha* (stalk) is called the *kalo*, and is considered a *makua*, parent plant. The younger shoots that grow from the *parent source* are called *'oha*, which is the root word for *'ohana*, meaning family. Kalani explained that as the plant is harvested, the *ha* is replanted and the generations of taro continue to flourish. As Kalani spoke, I realized the deep significance of this plant to the well-being of the people—not just dietary, but *spiritual*. The taro patches were replaced by sugar cane when the Islands were settled by foreigners. Far more than a change in crops, the enforced agricultural action was a direct assault, a direct heart attack on the *'ohana*—breath of life—of the Hawaiian people.

After sharing what I had learned from Kalani about the taro, Willie and I continued to talk about taro fields for the whole hour. Willie had a broad knowledge about the natural world and I knew it was a doorway into a deeper level of healing for him. Sometimes we don't realize that the stories we carry within our blood contain the medicine that can heal our wounded hearts. In Willie's case, his medicine was evident. He carried the stories, as passed on to him from many ancestors before, as well as stories he lived daily. Week after week we shared stories back and forth, some from my Jewish culture, mixed with my experience with Native peoples, and stories from Willie's Hawaiian culture and his life experience.

By this point, Willie had completely stopped drinking and his violent outbursts had ceased. He had even been able to resume hunting with his other brothers and uncles, something he could not do for months after the accident. Willie was clearly reconnecting to the magic of his own life.

As the weeks passed, Willie began to talk more and more about starting a taro patch in a large field by Annie's house. At one time the field had been used to grow taro, but for many years had only been used as a pasture for grazing animals. Finally, Willie decided that this was what he wanted to do . . . return the fields to taro. Perhaps it was Willie's personal memorial to his beloved brother Daryl. Although Willie knew this was a huge undertaking involving backbreaking work—clearing and leveling acres of land, planting each of the thousands of stalks by hand, monitoring the water levels daily—and his reward . . . the harvest . . . was a full year away after the initial planting, he set his task in motion with the help of his whole family.

When Willie told me that it takes one full year to harvest the taro, I remembered a story I had heard from a Rabbi, who said that at the time of a funeral when we are asked to throw a handful of earth onto the coffin, it is to symbolize the planting of the soul in Heaven . . . and that our mourning time lasts one full year. After that year, it is time to rejoin life to harvest the fruits of life.

In December, 1994, one year after the thousands of stalks had been planted, Willie, along with friends and family, harvested (pulled) their first taro. I was invited to participate and, of course, I was delighted and honored to accept. I bounded out of bed at 6:30 A.M., put on my black scrubby shorts and oversized T-shirt, and headed over to Annie's house for my first experience of pulling taro. With the sun still below the horizon, the pink-shaded mountains of peaceful Waimea Valley, the ever-present crowing of the roosters, and the croaking songs of the frogs, I stepped barefooted into the soft mud and knee-deep water, which provides the bed in which the taro plant takes root. The act of loosening the mother plant with my foot, reaching way down into the muddy waters with my hands and pulling out the taro, unexpectedly reconnected me to something I had been struggling with since our move.

I had desperately missed the many Native American rituals and ceremonies that I had participated in when I lived on the mainland. These rituals and ceremonies had connected me to a sense of the sacred within myself, to the feeling of belonging to something larger than myself. With no ceremonies to participate in since our move, I felt achingly disconnected from my relatives and the true melodies of my heart. I often felt lost and alone, with little to hold onto. Standing there in the taro patch that moist Kaua'i morning, holding the taro in my purple-stained hands, I remembered the story of the Milo tree and what Ray had told me. "When a tree like that is knocked down and you stand it back up and replant the roots, it becomes even stronger than before, because its roots have to reach deeper into the earth to get nourishment." For the first time since our move, I felt as if my roots had a place in which to plant themselves. Through this growing web of relationship with nature, the taro was clearly talking to me. In a sense I received a spiritual *heart transplant*.

As I pondered my new teachings from nature, the sound of laughter caught my attention. Glancing in its direction, I saw Willie and his family truly enjoying themselves, and I could not help but think about Daryl. Although I had never met him, I felt his presence and silently said, "*Mahalo* [thank you], for perhaps it is through your spirit that we are able to reconnect to our own breath of life."

There I stood with Willie, Annie, and their family . . . all of us up to our knees in water and mud, holding the taro roots in our hands, readying the stalks for the next planting. As I think about it now, it seems as if nature was telling us her own story about hope and healing, reminding us that in the cycle of life there is always a "next planting."

Steppingstone Nine

THE IDENTITY SHIELD

*When the shield is made visible it means: Here is the story. Enter into it
and be created. The story tells of your real being."*

—N. Scott Momaday[3]

*H*ave you ever found yourself wondering "Who am I? . . . I
don't even know myself anymore. My life feels like a big
blank to me." Well, I know I sure have, especially when I'm in the
midst of making major changes in my life. I guess that's why when I
come across something that can help me change my self-doubt into
self-appreciation, my ears perk up like a hungry little puppy's when
her name is called for dinner.

While teaching a workshop on the use of story, ritual, and ceremony for healing at the Warm Springs Tribe in Oregon, I had an
intriguing discussion with Art McConville, a Native American who is
an educator, artist, and spiritual leader from the Nez Perz tribe. After
sharing the Dreaming Pot story (see pp. 18–19) with him, Art told

me it reminded him of how he uses shields in his work with troubled adolescents to help them reconnect to their own identities in a positive way.

Art told me that, a long time ago, Native peoples used shields for different purposes; for example, in battle for protection or to identify who lived in each lodge. He said that rather than an address—such as 426 S. Elm Avenue—which tells us nothing about the person or family within, each lodge had a shield decorated with feathers, animal fur, shells, and other natural elements. In essence, these symbols told the story of who lived within the lodge or tipi.

After we spoke, I began to think about using the concept of shields in my work. Like the Dreaming Pot, my hope was to provide a creative experience that would help each person identify and reconnect with those symbols that best represented him or her . . . to identify and reconnect with who truly "lived within"—not with words, but with pictures—the oldest form of storytelling.

Since then shields have become an integral part of my personal life as well as of my professional training and speaking programs. I invite you to create your own Identity Shield in two ways. You can use the drawing of the circle provided on page 112, or you can follow instructions for creating a shield from real materials.

Drawing Your Identity Shield

Use colored markers, crayons, or whatever drawing materials you prefer.

1. Begin by closing your eyes and taking a deep breath, inhaling through your nose and exhaling through your mouth. After a moment or two imagine seeing the symbols that best represent

you—aspects of your life and personality in terms of nature, hobbies, and interests. The following questions can be helpful to you in identifying those symbols. Ask yourself:

- *What animal or bird most reminds me of myself?* I identify with the butterfly the most because of my interest in transformational change, as well as with the eagle because of my belief in the importance of vision. One of my colleagues thinks of himself as a bear because he likes to hibernate and is very protective. A young woman with whom I work identifies with a turtle. She says that when she is threatened, like the turtle, she seeks safety from within, while a teacher in one of my workshops identified herself as being most like a dolphin, loving the ocean and being very playful.

- *If I were a part of nature, what would I be?* Do you think of yourself as a strong tree with many branches, a mighty mountain with peaks and valleys, a gentle brook, a raging river, a powerful ocean?

- *What are your hobbies or interests?* A teenage girl with whom I worked remembered how much she loved being a photographer and drew a camera on her shield, while a psychologist in one of my workshops drew images of drums and a guitar because of his passion for music. Most touching for me was a time I was working with a woman in her seventies who was a double amputee. She decided to draw a picture of dancing slippers, because in her younger years she was a dancer. For her, the image reminded her of the dancer within who still had the ability to twirl and leap on the open stage of her mind.

With these questions in mind, let each symbol that best represents an aspect of your personality emerge in your mind's eye slowly and comfortably. Maybe only one image will come to you or perhaps many images will flow forward. It doesn't matter. As my Native American relatives say, "It is all good."

2. When the images are clear in your mind, open your eyes and begin drawing them within the circle of the Identity Shield.

My Identity Shield

Creating Your Identity Shield
With Real Materials

Another option is to make your Identity Shield out of materials, such as fabric or hide, bendable branches or basket weaving straw, paints, feathers, beads, and so on. This can be done by yourself or in a group situation. For example, the making of shields is an integral part of the retreats I co-lead for women as part of the Turtle Island Project. On these weekend journeys of renewal and healing, the women are given quiet time to wander in nature and reflect on where they are in their lives at that particular time, physically, mentally, and spiritually. The women are then asked to find a flexible reed-like branch along with anything else that "talks" to them from nature . . . anything they might want to be a part of their shield. We supply natural canvas cloth for the shield itself, acrylic paints of various colors, and a diverse collection of feathers, beads, and yarns.

After the women return from their self-reflective walk, with their branches and nature objects, they are shown how to bend the branches gently to form a circle. If need be, the branch can be soaked to provide more flexibility. When the hoop-like circle is formed, the ends are then fastened together with the yarn.

Next, they are asked to cut a circle from the canvas slightly smaller in size than the branch hoop. It should fit inside of the hoop art. Then they are shown how to fasten the circle of canvas to the branch hoop with the yarn in an over-stitch fashion.

The last step involves holding the blank shield in their hands, closing their eyes, taking a few deep breaths, and letting the symbols which best represent them emerge. When these symbols come to them, they open their eyes and decorate their shields.

We all work in one room and share stories, many spaces of quietness, laughter, song, and peace. It reminds me of the old quilting-bee circles I've seen portrayed in movies. Talk about naturalistic Team Building! Although many say there is no "I" in the word "team," I tend to believe that without the collective "I's" . . . the collective identities . . . there are no "eyes" for true vision. The key is to unite the identities by valuing the unique contribution and attribute of each person. This concept can be applied to families as well as business situations.

✻   ✻   ✻

After many years of working with shields, I have learned that each shield is dramatically unique to the individual at that particular time in his or her life and reflects strengths that may be obscured from his or her conscious view. For example, on the first retreat held in Arizona just after Hurricane Iniki in September 1992, my shield's center was blank. I could not come up with any symbols to represent myself. At first this disturbed me greatly, because symbols are an integral part of how I process information around me. As the weekend progressed, no matter how hard I tried to conjure up images, the canvas remained blank.

Finally, on Sunday morning, just after sunrise, I realized that the blank shield perfectly conveyed where I was at in that particular time of my life: I was literally *blank*. I had just moved away from everyone I knew, I had no job, no sense of spiritual connection, and had lived through a hurricane. My life was truly blank. It actually came as a relief to settle into, rather than resist, what I was experiencing. I was blank and numb and yet, at the same time, I knew that I was beginning again.

I keep this shield in a wicker basket, along with wild flowers I had picked that warm September weekend in Arizona, to remind myself of an old Taoist teaching I found in Lao-tzu's *Tao Te Ching*,[4] translated by Gia-Fu Feng and Jane English, about the value of empty space.

114

Thirty spokes share the wheel's hub;
It is the center hole that makes it useful.
Shape clay into a vessel;
It is the space within that makes it useful.
Cut doors and windows for a room;
It is the holes which make it useful.
Therefore profit comes from what is there;
Usefulness from what is not there.

Perhaps there have been times in your life when you also felt blank—devoid of ideas, feelings, or solutions to problems. Maybe as you make your own shield, you, too, will discover something important about the beauty of your usefulness and reconnect to the symbols of your personal heart-magic.

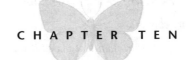

CHAPTER TEN

The Bowl of Light

"Above all that you hold dear, watch over your heart,
for from it comes life."

—Proverbs 4:23[5]

With straight, brown hair loosely dangling down the sides of her face, frail-looking Jaimi sat curled up in a bean-bag chair, separated from the other girls in the group. Everytime one of the girls spoke, Jaimi would roll her eyes as if to say, "Oh paleeeze," huff a bit, and stay securely curled up like a snail being approached by a potential predator. By the tender age of fifteen, Jaimi had wound up in gangs, a runaway, and covered her sad-

116

ness, anger, and feelings of hopelessness by cutting herself with pencil points and scraping her skin with paper clips. Like too many of our children today, Jaimi was a teenage girl who had been severely abused and neglected and bounced from foster home to foster home. Eventually, she ended up at the residential treatment center in Oregon that I visited every year between 1987 and 1995, where I worked with the children and staff using storytelling and rituals for healing.

On this particularly breezy Fall afternoon in 1993, we gathered in a large, cozy living room with overstuffed couches, big flower-printed floor pillows, and a few bean-bag chairs comfortably placed in front of a deep stone fireplace to *talk story* as we say in Hawai'i.

After an hour of interacting with the girls, they asked if I knew any good Hawaiian stories. After thinking a bit, I remembered an ancient Hawaiian story I found in the book *Tales of the Night Rainbow*[6, 7] as told by Grandma Kaili'ohe Kame'ekua to her grandchildren, Pali Joe Lee and Koko Willis. All the girls in the group gathered closer to hear the story . . . all except Jaimi. With arms tightly wrapped around her knees, she remained curled and distanced. Nonetheless, I began in the way that I best remembered the story.

Once a long time ago, there was this wonderful old Grandma who lived on the tiny Island of Moloka'i. Her name was Kaili'ohe Kame'ekua and she was over one hundred years old when she died in 1931. Grandma Kame'ekua and her family taught the children by stories, ancient chants, and parables. One story that was reeeally important to her 'ohana, which means "family" in Hawaiian, is that every child is born with a Bowl of Perfect Light. If the child takes good care of the Light, it will grow and become strong. The child will be able to do many things, such as swim with the sharks, and fly with birds, and the child will be able to know many things. However, sometimes there are negativities that come into a child's life . . . there are hurts, angers, jealousies, or pain. And these hurts, angers, or pain become like stones that drop into the bowl. And pretty soon there may be so many stones you cannot see the Light . . . and pretty soon the child can become like a stone; he or she cannot grow . . . cannot move. You see, Light and stone cannot hold the same space. But, what Grandma Kame'ekua tells us is that all the child needs to do is turn the bowl upside down and empty the stones and the Light will grow once more . . . Yes, the Light is always there.

When I finished the story, fourteen-year-old Mabel spontaneously said that she thought about her own abuse and use of drugs as a way of coping with her life's pains, struggles, and challenges. She said, "This bad stuff that happens is like the stones in the story. It just takes away the light." Sixteen-year-old Hannah said that she felt that the story talked about self-esteem . . . "like the bowl of light is like the pretty pockets we have inside us." I listened with an open heart as the girls processed what the story meant to each of them.

Many were visibly touched by this story, but I did not know how much the story touched one particular girl until a few minutes after the group had ended. It was Jaimi, the girl in the bean-bag chair. With her therapist by her side and with soft tears beginning to stream down her cheeks, Jaimi said, "Aunty Joyce, all my life all I ever see are clouds of darkness, but after hearing that story, a crack of light went through the clouds and I *know* that I am going to be all right." As Jaimi spoke, she used her shaking, pointed finger to draw in the air a crack piercing the darkness. Jaimi's gentle tears then released into strong sobs while she said that she had been suicidal and had just about given up hope of every being okay. Jaimi went on to say that all she ever felt was anger about the abuses she endured throughout her life, feeling like she was powerless to make the changes she needed to be happy. But when she heard the story, she knew that she could "empty the stones from my bowl," and most important, that there *was* a bowl of light for her.

Through her sobs, Jaimi's affect changed from hopelessness to determination. She decided that she wanted to make her own bowl of light out of clay and gather her stones, which would represent her pain, anger, and abuse. The light was clearly beginning to glisten through the darkness of Jaimi's life.

On a return visit about six months later, Jaimi was excited to show me the bowl she had made along with the many stones that she had collected. She invited me to go with her while she tried to find a place to empty her stones—literally. I felt honored to be included and agreed without hesitation. It was a delightfully moist Oregon day when we walked down the pine-tree-lined road that ribboned through the grounds of the treatment center. As we walked, Jaimi proudly told me about the changes in her life since first hearing the story: she was able to go to a regular high school, to make friends, and she was even able to go on a date. Chuckling a bit, she said, "I'd forgotten how good a Baskin Robbins hot fudge sundae is!"

Jaimi noticed a large boulder-sized rock nestled under the sweet-smelling pine trees and thought this would be a good place for her to empty her stones. After a few quiet, reflective, and prayerful moments, Jaimi carefully turned her bowl over, letting the many stones she had gathered cascade down the large rock onto the surrounding soft green grass. Jaimi then said, "Aunty Joyce, this is just like what that Grandma in the story said; kinda all we need to do is turn the bowl upside down, empty our stones, and the Light will grow again."

Jaimi is now in her twenties. She graduated from high school and wishes to continue her education. She met someone special and is expecting her first child. At last, Jaimi is living the dreams that had been locked away in the darkness of her despair.

When Jaimi and I last spoke, she told me that her bowl of light had been broken accidentally in a move. Feeling sad about what had happened, I suggested that perhaps she could make another one. Thoughtfully, Jaimi responded, "No, I don't have to do that, Aunty Joyce; my bowl of light is glowing inside of me and can never be broken . . . it's glowing in a different way."

Steppingstone Ten

BOWL OF LIGHT

"The story," the Bushman prisoner said, "is like the wind.
It comes from a far-off place and we feel it."

—Laurens van der Post[8]

Inspired by the ancient Hawaiian story, "The Bowl of Perfect Light," this steppingstone can help you rebuild and enhance a sense of self-esteem and self-appreciation . . . the hallmarks of both inner and outer success and well-being. As we saw with Jaimi, making her own bowl of light helped her to become an active participant in her healing process. When Jaimi decided to make her own bowl of light, she gave tangible expression to her inner changes . . . she created a living metaphor. The finished product wasn't shaped by anyone else's vision but her own. She also had to gather her own stones and decide when, where, and how to empty them.

Since hearing the story, I have included the making of a bowl of light in each of my workshops. In one of the high schools on Kaua'i, for example, I worked with a group of at-risk adolescents. After I told the story, I gave each teen a clump of fast-drying clay (about the size of a tennis ball) and showed them how to make their own bowls of light. I explained that they would need to let it dry overnight and then decorate it over the next few days. I also asked them to go to other classrooms and become storytellers by recounting "The Bowl of Perfect Light" to other students. As the teens shaped their bowls, they spontaneously started talking about their "stones," which were drugs, alcohol, and situations of abuse. By talking about their struggles in this way, they were already taking their first steps toward emptying the stones from their own bowls of light.

I don't know if Grandma Kaili'ohe Kame'ekua literally made her own bowl of light, but I do know that this story has inspired the birth of its tangible creation . . . and as it is with all births, growth follows.

Creating Your Own Bowl of Light

- You can use fast-drying, self-hardening clay (which usually comes in two-pound or five-pound boxes), acrylic paints, and brushes. Optional items include small objects gathered from nature, such as rocks, sand, leaves, flowers, or special trinkets that have significant meaning in your life.
- Next take a piece of the clay from the larger chunk and begin to shape it into a ball. While holding the clay ball, close your eyes, take a few slow deep breaths, and visualize your bowl.
- When you have the image in your mind, open your eyes and begin to shape the clay into your bowl. A helpful hint is to begin by poking an indented hole into the clay ball with your thumb and slowly form the bowl from that point, turning the

ball in your hand as you continue shaping from the center hole outwards.

- When the bowl is finished, let it dry overnight, or longer if possible.
- Next take out the art supplies and spread them out on a table, or if you prefer, you can work on the floor. Now take your dried bowl and again hold it in your hands, close your eyes, take a deep breath, and let the image of your bowl of light emerge in your mind's eye. Then open your eyes and begin to decorate your bowl.

I have often left my bowl unpainted, in its natural state. At other times, I have painted elaborate designs.

Drawing Your Bowl of Light

Another option is to draw your own bowl of light on the page provided. Just follow the simple instructions and enjoy . . .

- Take a few deep breaths, close your eyes, and imagine seeing your own Bowl of Light . . . its shape, colors, size, and so on.
- When you have the image, open your eyes, and draw it on the following page. Take your time and decorate it with all of the symbols that come to mind.

My Bowl of Light

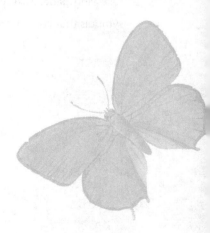

Identifying, Gathering, and Letting Go of Your Stones

The following questions can be useful in helping you identify your stones—the obstacles that block the inner light of your being and keep you from achieving your goals.

- What negative beliefs stand in the way of achieving my goals?
- What kind of life circumstances do I believe stand in the way of my success and happiness?
- What critical messages dampen my spirit? (Common examples include: "I'm not good enough." "I'm stupid." "I should just work harder." "I should just do more.")

Once identified, gather one stone for each obstacle. Next, take your time and decide how, when, and where you want to let them go. People sometimes say they aren't ready to let them go—they feel a need to hold onto them a bit longer. Respect your own timing. You will know when you are ready. However, if you feel you *want* to let them go, but something you can't identify seems to be getting in the way, perhaps the following questions can be helpful in clearing a path:

- What are the reasons I hold onto the stones instead of letting them go?
- What will happen if I let them go?
- What would my life be like without these obstacles?

Remember, letting go of your stones doesn't mean that the incident or experience never happened, it just allows you to reconnect to the light you were born with . . . your innate ability to appreciate yourself. The important message here is to respect your own timing. I always say to my clients, "You can't yell at seeds to grow." Healing and growth come from nurturance, guidance, and respect.

CHAPTER ELEVEN

Hidden Angels

"Sooner or later, in one lifetime or another,
each soul must accomplish its intended task."

—Rabbi Lawrence Kushner[9]

*B*a'shert in Yiddish means "meant to be." We have a higher destiny to our beingness other than just eating McDonald's hamburgers and accumulating credit cards. I often ask the kids with whom I work, "What do you think, God put you here just to steal cars and smoke dope?" That question usually percolates a laugh from an otherwise angry demeanor. It is also clear that our *higher purpose* is something that often reveals itself at the most unexpected times and challenging ways. For many of us, the road to fulfillment is never clearly marked or easily recognized. We are often jolted into discovery. Perhaps hidden angels are at work orchestrating the whole plan.

I met Ken Rutherford at the 1995 National Speakers Conference in Minneapolis, Minnesota. It was lunchtime and I was looking for a friend I was supposed to meet; however, I was unable to find her and decided to sit wherever there was an empty seat. The seat I chose was next to Ken. As the keynote speaker was being introduced, the audience offered a standing ovation. It was then that I saw that this handsome young man sitting next to me was an amputee. We all introduced ourselves when we were seated again. Ken and I struck up a conversation about our interests and speaking topics. He told me how he had lost his right leg in a land mine accident in Somalia while working to help the people there secure loans for their small business ventures. He was employed by the International Rescue Committee (IRC), one of the only sources of loans for small businesses in the war-ravaged country. Ken told me that one day while traveling down a dusty road on the way to an inspection of a lime quarry, the land cruiser Ken and his Somali aides were driving hit a land mine and was hurled into the air with such force that a three-foot-deep crater was gouged out of the road where the vehicle landed. With his right foot barely hanging by a piece of skin and his left foot badly abraded, Ken managed to drag himself through the pools of blood pouring out into the Somali dust to a radio, whereupon he was to call for help.

Since losing his leg, Ken's work has taken a new turn. He is currently attending Georgetown University to obtain a Ph.D. degree in International Relations and also devotes himself to land-mine legislation, where he hopes to have a dramatic impact on the global land mine crisis. He told me that an estimated 26,000 victims are maimed or killed in land-mine explosions throughout the world every year.

Later that evening while writing in my personal journal about meeting Ken, something unexpected happened to me. Memories of a very painful time in my life began to filter into my mind. At first I tried to push the memories away, thinking that they didn't belong. This was Ken's story, not mine. But the more I tried to ignore my thoughts, the more powerful their voice became, until I could no longer attempt to silence the strong memories that streamed forth. As it is with all stories, Ken's story became a steppingstone for me to walk upon as I crossed the personal rivers of my own life. I began to realize that while traveling down the road of expectant motherhood I, too, had been struck by a symbolic land mine many years ago.

In 1967, our first son was born prematurely, weighing three pounds eight ounces. Todd struggled for every breath he took from the first moments of his fragile life. This long-awaited time of joy was fraught with constant fear and uncertainty. Moment to moment my husband Eddie and I awaited news about Todd's dangerously rising blood count and irregular breathing patterns. Would he live? Would he die? Finally, after many fear-filled hours and prayer-filled days, Todd's elevated blood count became normal and his breathing more regular. He remained in an incubator in the intensive care section of the nursery for almost three weeks.

In those days, we could not hold him or feed him for the entire time he was in an incubator. Each day we watched through the nursery window as care was given to our little son by many loving nurses, until finally after four long emotion-spent weeks, we were able to take him home. . . . It was a true miracle.

Each month as he grew, I continued to feel that something was wrong with his development. I can't tell you why I noticed it—or *what* I noticed—because I had no training in child development at the time . . . no degrees other than my high school diploma and instinct. I kept mentioning my observations to the doctor, only to be told that I was just being an "overprotective mother" and not to worry. But my worry didn't go away, especially when all the other babies around us were beginning to sit, crawl, and walk. Todd did none of these activities in a normal way. He would sort of pull himself around with his arms. He would lean, not sit. His back was curved, not straight. Over and over I would ask the doctor what was wrong. Todd screamed all the time. What felt good to some children, like playing in the dirt, would set his temper tantrums flaring. Even when I picked Todd up to comfort him, he would thrash around and push himself away. Perhaps that was the most stabbing pain of all: My son was not comforted by my presence.

The more we tried to understand and question, the more our questions were sloughed off as parental nonsense, or answered by empty explanations like, "He's premature and it takes time to catch up." My worry soon turned to frustration, because I couldn't help my son. My frustration turned to anger. I knew my feelings were pulling me into the depths of my worst thoughts. Unable to control the turbulence of my reactions, I became an ugly, yelling machine. My pain over not being able to help my son, and of not being heard when I had asked for help over and over again, was turning me into a potentially abusing mother. Each day I would get up and pray for guidance and strength. Many days I would hide in my room so that I would not do anything to hurt my son. I was plummeting into an abyss of darkness. The more classes on parenting I attended, the more inadequate I felt, because nothing worked. I began to lose friends and, worst of all, I hated myself. How could I be a worthwhile woman and feel like I was the "mother from hell" at the same time? Although my husband was enormously supportive, he was unable to give me the answers that were not his to give.

Todd was now 18 months old and still not walking; he was not even sitting correctly. One of the specialists we had taken him to put him in a cast and said he'd be okay, his leg muscles were just twisted. Inwardly I knew something else was really the problem, but I didn't know what that something else was. When I questioned, my feelings were discounted once again. After all, who was I to question the head of orthopedics at one of Los Angeles's leading university hospitals. When the cast came off and Todd still wasn't walking—I was at the height of frenzy. It was then I was referred to Dr. Arnold Zukow,[10] "Dr. Buddy" as he is affectionately known to all his patients. It was his empathetic willingness to listen and a subsequent referral that lead us to the discovery that our son wasn't walking not because of a twisted muscle—but because of cerebral palsy.

Over the next few years, we were involved with extensive physical and occupational therapies to help our son. However, in the 1960s there was little, if any, recognition of the feelings parents experienced when they found out their child's handicap. All that we were exposed to were the false television programs that portrayed the "perfect understanding family." I had no place to go with my real feelings of anger, fear, and grief. My despair was deepening. I kept asking for help, but the answers I received from the professional community involved taking more parenting classes . . . classes that did not address the feelings of helplessness and loss I was experiencing on a daily basis.

I remember thinking, "What did I do wrong?" I thought that I was doing everything right when I was pregnant—going to a good doctor, taking vitamins, eating right, no smoking or drinking. Just like Ken, I was traveling down life's road trying to do the best job I knew how. And like Ken, what I didn't know was that my land mine was just up ahead . . . waiting to explode.

My long process of healing dragged me to the depths of pain

and feelings of failure. Like Ken, I, too, became verbally hurtful to loved ones around me as my feelings of despair deepened. And then, in 1971, more stones were placed in my bowl. I lost twin boys in my seventh month of pregnancy. The first little boy was born alive and died during the night. The second baby, who was stillborn, was wrapped in aluminum foil in front of me and carted away like a discarded piece of meat. I never got to hold or see either of them.

My hurt, pain, and rage continued to reach peaks and valleys. I was literally afraid of my own feelings. My husband stood by me, supportive and loving throughout these ordeals. However, my cries for help went literally unnoticed by the professionals I beseeched . . . until one day an astute nursery school director called and shared her concerns. I remember sitting in her office and feeling for the first time that someone other than my husband was hearing my "silent screams." She referred me to a new counseling program, the Julia Ann Singer Preschool Psychiatric Center, which focused on family therapy. In the early 1970s, that form of therapy was relatively new. At the time it was part of Cedars/Sinai Hospital, Thallians Mental Health Center.

I was also pregnant again and because of the dangers of losing this baby, too, I had to have a minor surgery and then remain in bed from my sixteenth week of pregnancy. Help had to be put on hold for just a few more months. With love and prayers our second son, Casey, was born healthy in 1972. After a few weeks of recuperation, we were ready to begin the program at the center.

From the first day of entering the program, I felt as if my cries were finally being heard. Perhaps this was the beginning of emptying the stones in my bowl. Therapy involved working along with therapists in the classroom, attending parent groups, and receiving family therapy five days a week for six intensive months. I began to learn that other parents felt as frustrated and pained as I did . . . that they, too, needed care and support as much as their special children.

Like Ken, my life took a dramatic turn. I was asked to volunteer at the center to work with other parents coming into the program. This opportunity led me into working directly with the parents in the weekly groups and finally being asked to participate in the intensive trainings offered to Master's and Doctorate level students.

At this point, I only had a high school diploma. Going back to school was the furthest thought from my mind—I didn't see myself as smart enough. (As a matter of fact, in junior high school I failed seven subjects on one report card.) But soon my interest in helping parents turned to a passion that was far more powerful than my educational fears. I devoured every bit of information I could find on working with parents who had children with various handicaps, or "life challenges," as they are called today. All the material I found focused on how special these children are, but the equally crucial reality—the full range of feelings a parent experiences—was dramatically simplified or left out entirely.

I remember sitting in a training session and trying to help students understand the frustrations the parents in our program were experiencing. I often used the following analogy. Imagine for a moment that your child gets a fever of 101. What do you do? Call the doctor and ask for help? Give your child Tylenol or aspirin or put the child in a tepid bath to bring the fever down? Let's suppose for a moment you do all these things and the fever still doesn't go down. In fact, it goes *up*. You get worried and call again. The doctor says to wait or bring the child in. And so you wait and wait . . . and finally after a long night, the fever finally breaks. How do you feel? Relieved . . . thankful. But let's suppose that, no matter what you do, your child's fever never goes away . . . it stays the same or even gets worse. You feel that no matter what you do, you will never make your child better. I explained that this was the *daily* experience and feeling of many parents of special-needs children. Many of the participants in the training group began to relate to these feelings of helplessness, frustration, and loss, and then shared their own personal experiences. Their empathy expanded from their work with the children to their work with the parents.

Although it remains true that each child brings his or her special uniqueness into this world and is loved for who he or she is, I do not know of any parent who wants his or her child to come into this world in a less than perfect fashion. We all count their little toes and fingers and wait to hear that our child is okay. We write all of their milestones in a baby book . . . remembering all of the firsts . . . first smile . . . first words . . . first step, and so on. I was no different. I wanted my baby to be healthy and perfect. It gave me no joy to record instead the dates of surgeries, casts, braces, and educational struggles.

As I began to become more vocal about my personal struggles, more and more parents in the groups with whom I spoke began to open up secret pockets of pain they carried within their hearts because of fear of rejection and shame. They shared how they would put on the "everything-is-perfect" smile and many times drank themselves into oblivion to kill the pain. However, I did not always get open acceptance for expressing my feelings. I also experienced criticism from those who wanted to perpetuate a perfect image of heroic parents overcoming all obstacles for their child, or perhaps they simply didn't relate to my type of experience.

I remember sitting in a producer's office pitching an idea for an ABC Afterschool Special that would address the parents' part of the struggle, in hopes of developing a story to help others who may have experienced similar feelings. After sharing my darkest moments, the program developer who was also present blurted out, "I don't get it. I don't get why you felt that way at all. I have a child who has reading problems and I don't feel that way." Her blunt, insensitive business tone told me that she really *didn't* get it, but at that particular moment in time, the old discounted feelings I had experienced so many times crackled through me like a bolt of lightning that precedes an impending storm. I thanked them both for their time and ended the meeting at that point.

Experiences such as this one only clarified my mission even more. I wanted to help other parents who shared in these despairing feelings in any way that I could. With encouragement, support, and love from my husband, family, friends, relatives, and colleagues, I went back to school, eventually getting a license as a Marriage, Family, and Child Counselor in 1978 and my doctorate in clinical psychology in 1982.

My dear son is now in his thirties. Through the years our relationship has endured the wrath of many hurricane-like storms, each time emerging with renewed strength, vision, and love. I believe that one of our greatest challenges in life is to continue to learn how to empty the stones that amass in our inner bowls of light. How do we do that? I am not always sure. What I am sure of is that each time our lives are graced by special people who openly share the life-challenging stories they have lived, we have the opportunity of reconnecting to a sense of Light . . . and perhaps to a feeling of hope. As Rabbi Kushner tells us when speaking about angels, "And so we understand that ordinary people are messengers of the Most High. They go about their tasks in holy anonymity. Often, even unknown to themselves. Yet, if they had not been there, if they had not said what they said or did what they did, it would not be the way it is now." Thank you, Todd, for being one of those hidden angels in my life.

Steppingstone Eleven

LIFE-STORY PUZZLE

"The craft of questions, the craft of stories,
the craft of hands—all these are the making of something,
and that something is soul."

—Clarissa Pinkola Estes[11]

The greatest legacies we have to give to our children are our stories. Each one is a piece to a great puzzle called our Life. In a poem addressing just such a subject, Rabbi Lawrence Kushner tells us, "Each lifetime is the pieces to a jigsaw puzzle. For some there are more pieces. For others the puzzle is more difficult to assemble."

When my mother died, I realized that I didn't know many of the stories that were part of her life. I knew some of them, but there were many missing pieces. She probably thought they were not very interesting. But what I have come to learn as a storyteller is that stories help us become whole in a fragmented world. Stories are neither good nor bad, they just are. Some contain elements of tragedy, while others contain experiences of joy. As it is with all puzzles, every story is made up of the sum total of its parts. One piece is not more important than the next, as they all must interlock in order to reveal the total picture. And the total picture is whom we are at the time. As we age, our puzzle grows, evolves, and expands.

Creating your Life-Story Puzzle is a steppingstone that will allow you to see each aspect of your life as an important piece that adds shape and substance to your own unique story.

- Begin your puzzle by writing down on a blank piece of paper any personal experiences that are important to you. Those experiences can be memories, accomplishments, struggles, goals, or values.
- Next, take a large, blank sheet of paper (perhaps poster paper) and color markers or crayons and begin to draw symbols representing each of those aspects . . . each of those experiences. The symbols do not need to be in any sequential order. For example, you may have had to go through personal struggles such as a surgery or experienced the loss of a loved one. You may also have children, a mate, friends, and a strong spiritual belief in your life that brings balance and joy. All of these aspects can be individually and symbolically drawn. You don't need to be an artist. Splashes of colors, shapes, stick figures, and line drawings are just fine. The symbols only need to make sense to you.

  For example, when I was a little girl of about seven years old, I sang and danced in Carnegie Hall. The symbol representing that experience that came to my mind was a pair of ballet shoes. As I look at the drawing of those pink-satin toe shoes, many memories stream forward into my consciousness, like the subway train rides I took with my mother from the Bronx to

Manhattan every Saturday in order to practice for the recital. It was our special time together, as she was a single mother in a time when it was very unfashionable to be one. She worked every weekday in a hat factory, so our time together was very special to me.

- Once you have drawn the important symbols on your page, draw interlocking lines around each of them in much the same way that pieces to a puzzle are shaped. Next cut out each piece so that they are all separated. Notice how you feel as you look at each piece, remembering that each one is an aspect of your own unique story.

- Finally, take your time to fit the pieces back together. Take a few reflective moments and look at the whole picture. Notice what you experience as you look at this picture.

This steppingstone is a wonderful experience you can share with your family. Each member can make his or her own Life-Story Puzzle regardless of age. Feel free to keep the pieces together, or perhaps place the pieces in a special container and from time to time, take them out and put the them together once again. As life presents new challenges and experiences, you may want to add to your puzzle or change it in some way that is meaningful to you.

CHAPTER TWELVE

Restocking Your Shelves

"The mind can go in a thousand directions.
But on this beautiful path, I walk in peace.
With each step, a gentle wind blows.
With each step, a flower blooms."

—Thich Nhat Hanh[12]

While relaxing on one of our golden sand beaches in Kaua'i, my husband and I were going over the stock in the little angel shop we decided to open just a few years after the Hurricane Iniki disaster. As we were talking about what to order and reorder, I innocently commented on how the shelves were looking empty and how important it was to keep our shelves stocked. I said that "People just don't feel good coming into a shop when the shelves are empty." Suddenly, I realized something about myself . . . *my shelves were empty*. And that was Empty with a capital E. Since the hurricane, I had been working nonstop with the children and families in the healing and recovery process. I was busy taking care of business, so to speak, and had little time just for me. It was a time of giving out energy constantly, with no time for personal exercise, eating right, attending nurturing workshops, or my soul's love . . . speaking and writing.

Since I am blessed with a lot of energy, I hadn't been paying much attention to my inner needs during this time. I thought I would be able to handle everything myself and keep on going and going and going like the Energizer Bunny from the battery commercials. I answered all of my mail and phone calls and balanced workshop requests and schedules, clients, husband, children, friends, and a counseling program. I was under this weighted blanket of illusion that I could handle it all, even though I wasn't sleeping well, I was gaining excessive weight, and my body felt like it might crumble from the pressure. Sound familiar?

It wasn't until that very moment of sitting on the beach and uttering the words "our store is looking empty, we need to *restock our shelves*," when I realized I was also talking about me. I didn't know whether to laugh or cry at this moment of awareness. My shelves were truly empty. Once I realized this, I began to think about what I needed to do to restock my shelves . . . my inner wellspring of Self . I began by making a list of all the things that I love doing: the "want-to's" not the "have-to's." I then circled the ones that were *the most possible* for me to do within the next week and wrote them in my datebook calendar, just as if I had an important appointment to keep. Of course, I did. The appointment was with my Self.

It has been some years since that fateful beach awareness day, and I am still reaping the rewards of my restocking decisions. Perhaps it was the inspiration of angels, whispering their message of self-care within the tropical breezes of our ocean.

Steppingstone Twelve

HOW TO FILL YOURSELF UP WHEN YOU'RE FEELING EMPTY

"If I am not for myself, who will be for me?
If I am for myself alone, what am I?
And if not now, when?"

—Hillel[13]

I feel that so many of us are in the same boat. The demands of everyday life and the pressures to keep up with its pace drain us of our soul's vitamin supplement . . . nurturing time for the self . . . and it is this nurturing time that allows our inner shelves to remain stocked.

Suggestions for Restocking Your Shelves

1. Find a quiet time and make a list of all of your *doing-for-others* activities. Next, make another list of all of your *doing-for-yourself* activities. Finally, look at both lists and see if they are balanced.

If the doing-for-others list far outweighs your doing-for-yourself list, see what you can eliminate. Your willingness to let go of certain demands allows you to make room for new ideas and personal growth.

2. Create a *dream picture* for yourself, by drawing symbols of what you want to do for yourself in both your personal and business life. For example, in your personal life you can get a new hairdo or implement a workout program, and in your business life you can learn how to use a computer or attend that long-desired seminar. Of course, you need not limit yourself in any way

3. Walk out into nature and pick up a rock, leaf, or flower. Hold it in your hands, close your eyes, and mentally ask it to teach you something you need to know right now that can help you restock your shelves. Nature has a way of transforming the "I can't do it mind" into the "all things are possible mind."

4. Take a *mini-mind vacation*. The following meditation exercise can help you feel renewed and refreshed so that you can have the energy and sense of well-being to face the demands and adventures of the day.

Mini-Mind Vacation

We all have times in our lives when we just want to get away from it all because of daily demands, pressures, and stress. Most of us are not in a position to just pick up and go on that desperately desired vacation. But we can *mentally* take a leave of absence, and enjoy a mini-mind vacation, in which we can regenerate our inner sense of well-being and personal energy. There are no suitcases to pack, no plane schedules to keep, and, best of all, it's *free*. Your passport and ticket are your innate ability to travel within your mind. You are the travel agent, pilot, navigator, and vacationer. So sit back and enjoy the journey.

First find a comfortable place either to sit or to lie down. Loosen tight clothing. If you are in an office where others are around, you can just adjust your body comfortably in your chair.

Now begin by letting your eyes rest on one object in front of you. Leaving your eyes opened and focused on that object, take a slow deep breath, inhaling through your nose and exhaling through your mouth, just as if you were softly blowing on a feather.

Repeat this breathing pattern three times, inhaling through your nose, exhaling through your mouth. Notice any changes in your perceptions or sensations. For example, notice if what you are looking at is becoming slightly out of focus . . . or perhaps are you feeling a tingling sensation or a sense of warmth or coolness . . . or see if there are any other shifts or changes in your awareness. These changes are letting you know that you are altering your state of consciousness from *outside busy thinking* to *inside peaceful being.* You may want to keep a notepad handy and write down your personal awarenesses. By doing so, you can become better acquainted with signals of shifts in your body and mind.

Now repeat the breathing exercise, once again focusing your eyes on a special object, taking slow, deep breaths, inhaling through your nose and exhaling through your mouth. With each breath, imagine that you are inhaling positive, comforting images and thoughts . . . maybe a place in nature or the presence of a loved one . . . and exhaling things you want to let go of in your life . . . any stresses, worries, fears.

After this set of three breaths, close your eyes and let your mind wander to a place you enjoy. Perhaps it's the beach, the mountains, the desert, or some other place that you have been to or wish to visit . . . a place that brings you comfort, happiness, a sense of well-being. Now take a moment to give this place a code name or word . . . a word that engenders a positive image or feeling. (For example, one of my comfort spots is located in the Koke'e mountains of Kaua'i. I have given that place the code word *fresh.* As soon as I say that word to myself, the image of that place in the mountains comes into my mind and, almost immediately, I feel the comfort of being there.)

Continuing to breathe easily and comfortably, enjoy exploring this place for a few long and luxurious moments. . . . Take the time to see the things around you that you enjoy looking at . . . noticing colors, shapes . . . the sounds that bring you pleasure . . . the fragrances and tastes that please you the most. You may even notice a special something that you want to reach out and touch . . . maybe it is a rock, a shell, a flower, or something else that reminds you of this special vacation . . . very much like a souvenir or photograph you treasure.

Take that special souvenir and tuck it away someplace inside of you, maybe a place within your body that needs to relax or receive a special message of comfort. . . . Enjoy exploring this place for a few more moments, then take one or two additional breaths, open your eyes slowly, and return to full comfortable awareness. Know that whenever you want to be reminded of the feelings of comfort and relaxation you experienced on this mini-mind vacation, all you need to do is take another slow deep breath and repeat the name you have given this vacation spot; it is your unique resort with unlimited resources for expansion and discovery.

Remember to take the time to **RESTOCK** YOUR SHELVES and fill yourself up when you're feeling empty. By doing so you can

Reach for your goals

Enjoy an aspect of nature each day

Seek new ventures

Treasure your uniqueness

Open your heart to love

Create beauty within your surroundings

Kindle your dreams

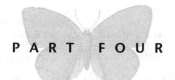

PART FOUR

Rituals and Ceremonies for Remembering What Deserves to Be Cherished

"The more materialistic science becomes, the more angels shall I paint; their wings are my protest in favor of the immortality of the soul . . . "

— E. C. Burne-Jones to Oscar Wilde (1880)[1]

*I*n this part of the book, I deal with illness, death and dying—subjects most of us want to avoid. We usually do not think of reconnecting to the magic of life in relation to illness or death. However, the stories I relate illuminate a path past the painful realities of illness and death to those dimensions of living that contain humor, determination, and courage.

The steppingstones here will show you how to reconnect to a sense of joy in your life, to transform everyday occurrences—such as the rising and setting of the sun, drinking a glass of water, or taking a bath or a shower—into rituals or ceremonies for honoring life and letting go of worries. In addition, I give you suggestions on how to create rituals and ceremonies for healing and celebrating numerous aspects of your life's personal journey.

I present each story and steppingstone as a tribute to those angels who take flight from this world, leaving us with the courage to grieve, the gift of memory, and the magical quality of cherishing life.

CHAPTER THIRTEEN

Angels of Flight

"What is important? The answer is Love."
—Gershon Adolphus Tucker III[2]

When I began to write this story, I thought it was going to be about Gershon, a young man, in his last weeks of life battling AIDS, who asked the impossible of his older sister, Charlee—to take him to Disney World. However, as I listened to Charlee's account of her very painful and often humorous experiences with Gershon, I became more and more convinced that this story would not be about Gershon and that wish-fulfilled trip as much as it would be about the importance of what his life stood for . . . joyful living. What is joyful living? A story told to me by Dr. Richard Crowley, my close friend and colleague, perhaps best describes its meaning.

When Richard was in Bali on a sabbatical, he came upon a small town in which a gathering was taking place. The gathering was led by a Zen Buddhist priest. It seemed that the day before, the people had asked the priest to tell them his secret for finding happiness daily. The priest told them to come back the next day and he would share what he knew. Richard joined the group and looked forward to learning the secret.

The priest sat on a slightly elevated platform, and had a medium-sized, plain brown bag next to him. The group waited in curious silence as the priest reached inside the bag and took out a black, rotten banana. The priest then held it up in plain view for a few long moments and said, "The Past." After putting the rotten banana down, he reached inside the bag again and this time pulled out a hard, green banana. Holding it up for the group he said, "The Future," and once again he put the banana down on the small table next to him. Finally, the priest reached his hand into the bag once again and this time took out a firm, ripe, yellow banana. He peeled back the skin slowly and then took a bite of its sumptuous center. After swallowing what he had eaten, he looked at the group and said, "The Present."

When I heard this story, I could not help but think of its simple, but powerful teaching. Most of us spend so much time contemplating the mistakes or missed opportunities of the past or worrying about what's going to happen that we forget about the present moment. We forget that the present is truly all that we have. We forget how to eat from the ripe banana. We must remember to get nourishment from the fruits of today.

As I listened to Charlee describe her experiences with Gershon, I knew he was someone who truly ate from the ripe banana. He loved life and embraced its daily challenges with a sense of purpose and joy. Even in his most difficult and weakened time on earth, his desire was to experience joy. As a graduate of the London Academy of Music and Dramatic Art, Gershon's greatest love was Shakespeare. Charlee said that a few months before Gershon died, he contemplated the famous soliloquy "To Be or Not to Be" in relation to his life-threatening situation. He kept talking about it in terms of "should he be in life, or not be in life?" Finally, Gershon became clear. While he was still living, he was going to live life to the fullest.

Gershon talked about the *dis-ease* in his body as being something he would accept, but it would not keep him from *living* the joys of life. One such joy was the love affair he had with Disney World ever since he was a little boy. He was especially fixated on roller coasters. In December, just a few months before he died, Gershon decided he wanted to visit Disney World and ride the roller coaster one more time. The doctors and hospital staff began arranging it. At first, Charlee didn't believe the doctors were *really* going to go through with his request. She thought the doctors were doing something to help their parents accept his death. Charlee even flew across the country to try to talk the doctors out of it. She kept thinking to herself, "This is just crazy. Gershon is so frail, how can he make such a trip?" When Charlee was about 30,000 feet in the air, something she describes as unexplainable changed her mind. Perhaps it was the whispering of angels, like a wake-up call. Charlee realized that, of course, he would go . . . and even more than that, she would go with him. At first Gershon said that he was going with his friend, Artie. When Charlee heard this, it was like a call to action. "That was my brother . . . what if he died on the trip and no family members were around to be with him?"

The preparation for the trip was tremendous. Charlee and Artie went through two solid days of intense emergency training, in which they learned how to administer infusions and medicines and care for his personal needs. Gershon was given transfusions that contained steroids so that he would be strong enough to live through the trip. Although the doctors and hospital staff were excited about this trip, Charlee became increasingly frightened. She remembers that as Gershon was wheeled on a gurney to the plane, she put all her faith in God and kept praying, "Dear God, please don't let him die on the plane. . . . Please let me be able to handle it. Please help me." Charlee was sure that God heard her prayers and sent angels to be with them every mile of the way. Finally, after what seemed like endless hours in flight, they quite literally landed safely on a "wing and a prayer."

There are many moments Charlee remembers about the trip. One in particular stands out. Earlier that day Gershon's mood swings began to exacerbate. He especially lashed out at Artie to such a point that Artie left them for a while and went off by himself. That same day, Gershon was determined to go on the Runaway Train ride. This ride carries many warnings to its passengers. Charlee became terrified. Although she knew it was one of his last wishes, she was also aware that her brother was becoming increasingly weak. At the last minute, the person at the gate told him that he just couldn't go. Gershon begged and said he could make it. With spindly arms, he desperately tried to stand to prove it to him, but he was just too weak. He couldn't go. For both Charlee and Gershon this was a tormenting moment of face-to-face confrontation with the reality of his physical impairments. Charlee remembers her tears mounting as she wheeled Gershon through the crowded park.

After a short time they came upon the Pirates of the Caribbean, a ride that didn't demand anything more than sitting and watching the fun-filled sights. Both of them decided this would be a ride they could go on without the threat of danger. As it turned out, this was one of the hardest but one of the most important experiences she shared with her brother, for there in the darkness, she was able to let her tears flow freely. She was grateful for the closeness that she shared with her brother, but saddened by the fact that he couldn't go on the ride that he came for—the Runaway Train.

I find it amazing that both rides provided a metaphor for their plight. Gershon's battle with AIDS was like a runaway train, an illness that uncontrollably ravaged his body. On the other hand, Pirates of the Caribbean provided an adventure that is entered in darkness but results in an emergence into light. After Pirates of the Caribbean, Charlee and Gershon embraced and clearly felt better about what had happened and about their relationship. Later on, Artie caught up with them and also felt better about their earlier struggles. By the end of the day, Gershon realized that he had had enough and was ready to go home. A few weeks later on April 21, 1993, Gershon Adolphus Tucker III died in his parents' home.

On the Easter Sunday before his death, Charlee remembers a magical moment that stays forever etched in her heart. While she spoke to him, she recognized his true Spirit. There were clearly "two beings, one body and one soul, two energies dancing in his eyes." She knew at that moment that she was ready to let him go. She even told him that "we're all ready now, whenever you're ready to go, you can go. We'll be just fine." But Gershon never lost his sense of humor even at the end. His response to her was, "I'm not goin' anywhere yet."

As I think about it, there are many kinds of angels. There are angels in heaven, living with God and doing those things that can only be carried out from above, and then there are angels who live here on earth, helping us to accomplish our most difficult tasks and helping us to reconnect to the magic of living. Charlee is one of those earth angels. I'm sure that Gershon knew that when he asked her to take him to Disney World. One angel always recognizes another.

A dear friend of both Charlee's and Gershon's, Matt Nolen, sculpted and glazed small, cylinder-shaped cups engraved with the words "Don't Postpone Joy," and gave them as gifts to those present at Gershon's memorial service. Could it be that Gershon found the *Angelic Internet* and passed this message on to each of us still living on earth through this gift? Charlee gave me one of these treasured cups and it sits on a shelf above my desk next to her picture. Sometimes when life feels overwhelming for me and I think I have to accomplish, accomplish, accomplish—when I feel tethered by the worries of the future or get seeped into the memories of the past—I look up and see the words "Don't Postpone Joy," and I am reminded of what is *really* important.

Steppingstone Thirteen

MY CUP OF JOY

*"Go to your fields and your gardens, and
you shall learn that it is the pleasure of the bee to
gather honey of the flower, But it is also the pleasure
of the flower to yield its honey to the bee."*

—Kahlil Gibran[3]

*E*ach morning I slowly meander into the kitchen and fix my
wake-me-up cup of coffee. Mmmm, the smell of freshly brew-
ing coffee fills the air as I watch, somewhat impatiently, as the rich,
dark liquid begins to drip through the filter into the glass pot. I then
pour that first cup and sip slowly, enjoying the rich taste as it goes
down. For me, it is a cup of pure wake-up joy. As I think about it,
wouldn't it be nice to begin and end each day sipping from a cup filled
with joy? Perhaps it could lead to another kind of wake-up feeling.

How many times do we rush through our day not even thinking
about the gifts we may have received that day . . . gifts that fill our
inner cup of joy? Perhaps it was a smile from the supermarket check-

out person or a hug from your child. Maybe it was a kind note from a colleague at work letting you know that you did a good job on a project or perhaps you received a phone call from a friend or relative you hadn't heard from for a long time. Most of the time these simple gifts go unnoticed and we remain focused on what's not going well.

This Steppingstone is meant to remind you to reach for your cup of joy each day and to decide what is in it or what you want to fill it with. Find a quiet place, take a deep breath, and ask yourself the following questions. The answers may come to you in the form of thoughts or images. Write them down in the space provided below. Use additional paper if you so desire.

- What gives me joy in my life?

- With whom do I feel full, respected, joyful?

- What would I like to be doing in my life that I am not doing? In other words, what joy am I postponing?

- Next, look at the answers to these questions and ask yourself, What am I willing to do that will bring joy into my life today?

- The next step is simple . . . Just do it!

CHAPTER FOURTEEN

Susana

> *"Music is well said to be the speech of angels."*
> —Thomas Carlyle[4]

Whenever I hear the song "You are my sunshine, my only sunshine . . ." I can't help but think of my dear friend Susana who died about ten years ago. There we were, tooling down Camelback Road in Phoenix on our way to a Mardi Gras carnival, made-up to the hilt with glittering eyes, red painted lips, and brightly colored clothing. No one would have suspected that

Susana only had a few months more to live. As we sang "You make me happy when skies are gray . . . " I tried to push away thoughts of the inevitable. I didn't want to lose my friend, this woman I had come to think of as my sister, in such a short amount of time. But then again, I am beginning this story near its end, so I'd better begin at the beginning.

I met Susana at a retreat on Native American perspectives of healing in 1987. From the moment we met, we shared a special feeling of familiarity. Susana was all of four feet ten inches tall, small-framed and bouncy, with a Spanish-sounding accent that was song-like to my ears. Her eyes were wide and coal black, glistening with awareness.

We loaded her van with all the camping gear and off we went for a weekend adventure . . . and what an adventure it was! It was my first experience with Native American people and I didn't know what to expect. All I knew was that I wanted to be there.

During one of the ceremonies, a "talking circle," Susana revealed that she had been diagnosed with cancer of the colon and was deciding whether or not to have surgery. This was the first time I had heard her talk about her illness. I remember looking at her in disbelief. Her enormous zest for life and glowing positive spirit left no room in my mind for doubt. I thought to myself, "This lady is absolutely going to be okay."

After the talking circle, we gathered wood for a fire. I still remember Susana picking up a heavy axe and swinging it over her head and down onto a large log over and over again, saying, "This is my cancer . . . this is my cancer." I ran and got my camera to capture this Kodak moment in a snapshot. We both laughed and talked every moment we spent together. By the end of the weekend, our bond was clear. We were sisters.

Over the months that followed, Susana made a decision not to have surgery but to embark instead on alternative healing approaches.

Although Susana knew the possible outcome, she believed that she had the ability to heal and that there was a purpose to this illness.

Month after month her pain grew worse, but she still did not want to go through any surgery, until she had to undergo an emergency colostomy for an obstructed bowel. During the surgery, her doctors discovered that the cancer had spread to her liver.

It was midday on a Friday when I was picked up at Sky Harbor Airport in Phoenix, Arizona, by Cristina Whitehawk, a special friend who was one of many earthly angels who had been caring for Susana and her four children since the surgery five weeks earlier. As we entered Susana's apartment, I inwardly gasped, for there she sat weighing all of seventy-four frail pounds, slumped in an oversized recliner by the sliding glass window in her living room. Her face was paste white, her voice was weak, and hollow darkness surrounded her once-glowing eyes.

My heart shuddered as I rushed to her side. Almost immediately Susana began to cry, saying how nauseous she was, how much pain she was in, and how she didn't want to go on living this way. As I knelt down by her armchair, I asked Susana if she would feel like living if the nausea and pain could stop. Susana responded with an unequivocal YES! "Okay then, would you go along with me while I teach you a little self-hypnosis?" She squeezed my hand and once again said "Yes." I continued to hold her hand and said, "Good, then begin by focusing your eyes over there, and take a nice slow deep breath, in through your nose and out through your mouth . . . and after three slow breaths, close your eyes and just let yourself drift to a special place you would like to visit. . . . " I asked Susana to signal me by lifting a finger to let me know when she was in that special place. In a few moments the tension lines on Susana's forehead and around her mouth relaxed and her breathing transitioned from quick and shallow to a slower, deeper rhythm. I waited as the little finger on her left hand lifted slightly. While she was in a light trance I talked to

Susana about endorphins and how the body knows just how to bring comfort when we need it. Susana spontaneously whispered, "Endorphins are like dolphins." With a slight smile appearing on her face, Susana said, "I will name my dolphin Onie. . . . Onie will be my helper."

As I wanted to build upon Susana's awareness, I continued to intersperse suggestions for comfort with stories about dolphins for approximately twenty minutes, at which time Susana opened her eyes, looked around, and said with a lilt of surprise in her voice, "My nausea . . . it's gone . . . it's gone for the first time in the five weeks since my surgery." We all smiled in validation of her accomplishment. Cristina then hung a large, hand-made sign on the wall that read,

> As a woman desires, so she wills.
> As she wills, so she becomes.
> As she becomes, so she is.

Susana readjusted herself in her chair and to our surprise blurted out, "Let's go shopping, Joyce. I want you to fix us Shabbat dinner (Shabbat is a sacred time of the week in the Jewish tradition honoring the Sabbath) of chicken soup, matzo balls, roasted chicken and potatoes, the whole works!" This was the first time in five weeks since Susana's radical surgery that she had the energy to go anywhere, let alone shopping. Although she was still visibly weak, a strength inside of her began to flower. As we wanted to support her blossoming glow, Cristina and I said, "Well, what are you waiting for, let's get ourselves dressed." After she slipped into a colorfully printed over-sized dress, Susana was even up for makeup.

When we returned from the store with bundles galore, the cooking began. The smells permeated the apartment and each of Susana's children arrived home. It was also one of her sons' birthday and Susana's dear friend and companion, David, called to tell us that he'd pick up a cake on his way home from work.

David is a unique man who helped Susana in any way that he could, including being a surrogate father for the children. David slept on a lounge chair in the living room, woke up to change Susana's IV, and tended to her bed needs each night. He was up early in the morning to help get the children off to school and then would go to work. He was not her husband or her lover, as we commonly understand the word; he was a friend whose heart stretched the word well beyond its meaning.

The table was set and we were all seated. I asked Susana to light the Shabbat candles and then I taught her and the children the prayer: "Ba-ruch, A-tah a-don-nai eh-lo-hey-nu me-lech ha-o-lam asher kid-sha-nu b'mitz-vo-tav v'tzi-va-nu l'had-leek nair shel Shabbat. Amen." ("We thank you God, guide of the world, who helps us feel holy when we light the festival lights. Amen.") We then recited prayers for the wine and bread. We were moved and grateful to be together . . . especially because this would probably be the last birthday Susana would have with her son.

Susana ate a whole bowl of chicken soup with a matzo ball as well as noodles, chicken liver, bread, and two glasses of kosher wine. She was feeling better. We all laughed as her son opened his presents and told jokes, as only a fourteen-year-old can.

Later that evening Susana's nurse came and hooked up her IV. With compassion and gentleness, the nurse showed me the intricacies of what to pay attention to on the monitor and how to hook and unhook each needle change. While my conscious mind was completely riveted to each detail, I could feel a numbness creeping through my insides as I tried to learn this procedure. I wrote down each step of the instructions so that in the middle of the night, I would have them as a guide. I truly did not trust my memory.

The nurse left and David decided to stay as support in case I ran into any difficulties. It was my first night with Susana and I was frightened. I thought to myself, "I am not a nurse or a physician. What would I do it something went wrong?" Within fifteen minutes of the nurse's departure, Susana called my name in a frail and pain-choked voice. "Joyce, I'm sorry, but I need to go to the bathroom." I took out my list of what-to-do-and-how-to-do-it instructions and began to unhook her IV, reattach the new needle, and help her to the bathroom just some twelve feet away. Since Susana was a very private person, she closed the door and a few seconds later I heard the bath-tub water running. "Are you alright?" I asked, as I waited outside by the door. Her little daughter was right by my side, sucking two of her fingers. The water stopped and Susana replied, "Yes, I think so. The only way I can urinate is in the bathtub sitting in warm water. I pass big blood clots when I urinate and this helps with the pain." *Blood clots!* This was the first time I had heard about this particular ordeal. After a few long minutes of waiting, Susana's pained voice changed into one that reflected relief. "You can come in now, I passed it," she said.

When I opened the door, I couldn't believe my eyes. For there sat my dear friend in a bathtub of blood, which was slowly draining . . . and lying between her pale, spindly legs was a clot the size of a large fist. My heart pounded with fear as I leaned over to help her out of the tub. As I wrapped Susana in a towel, she told me this had been going on since she had left the hospital. The doctors treating her said it was "normal" for this stage of her cancer. Rather than discuss the absurdity of this kind of insensitive response, I just let it go for the rest of the evening and helped her into bed.

This routine of hooking and unhooking her IV, visiting the bath-room, and holding her continued throughout the night. In the morn-ing Susana told me that she felt as if she had been abandoned by her doctor. He had told her he couldn't help her anymore and had stopped calling to check on her. As she spoke about her feelings, she

160

changed from tearful to angry. I asked if she had expressed this anger to him directly and suggested it might be a good time to do so. Susana said that she hadn't and immediately asked for the telephone. I sat next to her as she spoke. Once again, when she told him about the clots, he responded that he couldn't help her because she was in the final stages of her illness. With strength in her voice, Susana blurted back, "I'm not dead yet. I want a doctor to work with me while I am *still alive . . . I am still living.* If you want to work with me with that in mind, I would like that, but if not, please refer me to someone who would." Her face remained strong as he responded by saying, "Then I will refer you."

I couldn't believe what I was hearing. Susana hung up the receiver and said, "Now I know what I have to do . . . I have to find a different doctor." Her voice was strong and determined. We called Dr. Carl Hammerschlag, a dear friend, a psychiatrist, and a colleague whom we knew shared a vision of healing that involved healing the spirit as much as healing the body, and explained the crisis situation to him in detail. At this point Susana was not going to back down. She was going to find a new physician no matter what it took. Hearing the strength in her voice, Carl immediately got on the case and contacted Dr. Howard Silverman,[5] who agreed to become her primary-care physician. Susana seemed to come alive after this decisive change. With a twinge of twinkle back in her eyes she said, "Joyce, there's a carnival here tonight, a Mardi Gras. Let's go." I couldn't believe my ears. Just eight hours ago, she was barely able to move; now she was ready to embark on a major excursion.

Her little daughter was right by our side as we painted our faces with designs of all kinds. We searched for the brightest colored clothes, gaudy jewelry, and funny hats, and off we went, wheelchair and all. When we got to the park where the Mardi Gras was being held, Susana's eyes brightened. She wanted to eat everything there was, cotton candy and all. We played games like tossing little rings on Pepsi bottles, listened to the music that played over the loudspeakers, enjoyed the strolling entertainers who performed magic, juggled, and twisted long balloons into the shapes of elephants, dogs, and such. It was a night that rang with laughter, joy, and life.

On the way home, Susana said, "Let's sing my favorite song." Without hesitation the words streamed forth. "You are my sunshine, my only sunshine. You make me happy when skies are gray. . . . " On and on we sang, continuing our concert all the way home. It was the last time Susana and I shared such magic in this life. She died a few months later. But it was not the last time we shared magic.

Steppingstone Fourteen

"A monk once asked his master, 'No matter what lies ahead, what is the Way?' The master quickly replied, 'The Way is your daily life.' "

—Shoshitsu Sen XV[6]

We all recognize the rituals and ceremonies associated with rites of passage and holidays related to our particular religious and cultural beliefs. We spend endless hours preparing special foods, decorating our homes, and shopping for special gifts to celebrate or honor each occasion. In thinking about the above quote, coming, as it does, from a fifteenth century Zen tea master, I am also reminded of the importance of creating rituals and ceremonies in our daily lives to reconnect us to something beyond our material possessions and ourselves—to infuse us with a sense of community and the sacredness of all life.

The following two rituals can help you learn how to use water as a "medicine" to help restore and embrace a feeling of harmony and a sense of well-being. Just as a wilted plant needs water to restore its ability for healthy growth, so too do we need water to help us stay balanced when life presents its daily challenges. Both of these rituals were taught to me by Native American relatives. It is with their loving permission, and with the greatest honor and respect, that I share them with you.

Water as Life

Towards the final months of Susana's life she wanted to go to a Native American prayer ceremony. As it is with all miracles, they come when we least expect them, and an opportunity arose for us to attend such a ceremony. It was my first time in this kind of a ceremony and I was very conscious of not wanting to offend anyone, especially being the only white person in the tipi. Susana sat next to me as the chanting, prayers, and drumming continued throughout the night. During one particular time in the evening, one of the women brought a bucket of water into the tipi and began passing it to each person seated in the circle. At first I thought, "Oh, this is good, I am really thirsty. I could drink this whole bucket myself." I graciously took the cup that was handed to me and quickly dipped it into the plain metal bucket of water placed before me and brought it to my lips without hesitation. As I was about to take a sip, I noticed that the Native American man I now call Brother was shaking his head and under his breath he said, "Uh-Uh!" "Oh, great," I thought to myself. "The white kid over here is really messing up." He smiled and whispered, "That water is your life. How do you want to drink from it?" As he said that, something stopped inside of me. I thought about what he said: "That water is your life. How do you want to drink from it?" His words transformed a simple drink of water into a ceremony of life.

At that moment I held the same cup of water but with a far different feeling. I held it between both of my hands, rather than in just one hand, and closed my eyes for a few moments. When I opened them, I looked into the cup and then brought it to my lips slowly. The thirst I experienced earlier vanished and what remained was a deep sense of relationship to the water. It brought a feeling of renewal to me that I still embrace.

One of the Native elders helped Susana with the cup and encouraged her to drink as well. As the water passed through her lips, she was able to shift her body, even in its weakened state, and smile.

It seemed as though the water had awakened a sense of life in Susana's frail and withered body.

To this day when I go to take a drink of water, whether it is from a glass or from a water fountain, I remember the words shared with me that special night. As I drink, I think about my life. Depending on how I am feeling, I may take small sips, larger gulps, or drink it slowly.

That night I was also told that "Water is woman. It is the woman who prays over the water. It was the first medicine given to us by the Creator, because it is water that must flow first in order for a baby to be born." With permission from my Native relatives, I often tell this story to participants in my workshops and then have them break into smaller groups and sit in a circle. One member of the group holds a pitcher of water and gives each participant a cup. The pitcher is then passed clockwise in the circle to each person. He or she takes the pitcher and pours some water into the cup. There is no talking. It is a quiet time of self-reflection.

This water ceremony can become a ritual you use either for yourself, or you can share it with your families, friends, or even business colleagues who may be feeling overwhelmed by the demands of every-day life. No talking *has* to take place. However, if anyone who is par-ticipating wants to share his or her experience, encourage it. The story provides the seed from which the ritual develops . . . and the ritual provides a flower from which the fruit of self-awareness and relation-ship ripens.

Perhaps this would be a good time to experience this ritual for yourself. Just pour a glass of water, hold it in your hands for a few, long moments, take a deep breath and repeat to yourself, "This water is my life . . . how do I want to drink from it?" After you finish drink-ing your water, notice what feelings, sensations, or thoughts come to mind. If you wish to record these awarenesses, you can do so in writ-ten form, or you can draw them on the page that follows. Just as you may take a break and drink a cup of coffee or tea, take time to pour yourself a cup of water and renourish the sacred gift of your life.

Water Ceremony Awarenesses

A Bathing Ritual for Releasing Worries

Another example of how to use water for healing was shared with me by a woman from the Cherokee tribe. Jenny told me to think of bathing as a ritual for purification . . . a time for letting go of worries and concerns . . . not just a routine to keep me smelling good. I was familiar with the concept of bathing for purification since one of the rituals in Judaism is the *mikvah*, a bathing ritual in which women participate after birth or menstruation. Jenny's ideas are different in that it is not necessary to wait for any seasonal passage to enjoy this bathing ritual; instead it can become part of daily life.

Jenny suggests bringing special flowers or scents into the bathroom and perhaps lighting candles. By making these few simple changes, we can transform our ordinary bathroom into a sacred space. While you bathe, think about the things that may be troubling you, physically, emotionally, or spiritually, then cup water in your hands and release it over your body or whatever part of your body that may be needing comfort. After your bath (or shower), remain in the tub and watch until all of the water goes down the drain, taking with it all of your worries and concerns. In essence, you will create a *web of relationship* between the action of taking a bath and your mind, body, and spirit. The next time you take a bath or a shower, try these suggestions and notice how you feel afterwards.

CHAPTER FIFTEEN

Postcards From the Other Side

*"Angels are silent. They just are
there for you. It is like an inside thing."*

—Anonymous, Age 7[7]

When a loved one dies, we often wonder if there are ways he or she can communicate with us other than through his or her physical presence. Thousands of people have recounted personal stories in which they have received messages in many ways, such as through dreams, visions, fragrances, and moving objects, letting them know something important about their loved ones. Questions often arise as to whether or not these encounters are true or are they simply wishes people hold onto in order to ease the pain of loss. I do not have the answers to such questions; however, I have had my own experiences and it is these I share with you in this chapter.

A "Deer" Sister Message

One morning in San Diego, California, just one month after Susana died, we shared magic once again. As part of a three-hour workshop, I had been teaching a group of professional mental health care workers, physicians, nurses, and educators a breathing exercise (the one I had taught Susana) that is used for relaxation and as an induction for hypnotherapy. I directed the group to focus their eyes on one spot, take three comfortable breaths, and after the third breath, to let their mind travel to a place they would like to be. I told them to explore this place fully and to discover a souvenir they would like to bring back when they returned to full conscious awareness. And that's when I had one of those experiences that you may have read about in an Edgar Casey or Shirley MacLaine book.

After the group returned to full awareness, I asked, as I always do, if anyone wanted to share his or her experience. The group seemed calm and comfortable. Different people spoke of their personal feelings of calmness, relaxation, comfort, and so on. At one point I noticed a woman sitting in the front row with a lovely soft expression on her face and I asked if she would like to share her experience with us. Patricia happily agreed.

As Patricia took a deep breath, she had found herself sitting on the balcony of her home in Sedona, Arizona. She had heard a call of some kind and put out her right arm. A great white eagle flew to her and landed on her arm. The eagle plucked a white feather out of its wing and placed it in her mouth. Patricia took the feather from the eagle and tucked it within some kind of deer-like fur that surrounded her body.

Then the eagle turned her head and looked at Patricia in one eye and then in the other, circled, and flew off. Patricia said she saw the eagle fly away and felt as if she had been left with a cloak of feathers that came up over her head. She said she came back into the room as if she was the eagle.

As Patricia ended the recounting of her experience, I was intensely aware of chills running electrically through my body. I told the group that I knew that this was not the agenda for the workshop, but that I felt compelled to respond to Patricia's experience. The group was more than eager to hear more. I went on to say that just a month and a half prior to this workshop, a dear friend of mine had died of cancer. Susana was a spiritual woman and deeply involved with Native American teachings. A few months previous to her death, Doctors Carl Hammerschlag and Howard Silverman, along with many Native American people, sponsored an all-night prayer meeting for Susana attended by her children, many friends, and health-care workers. She was surrounded by the most powerful medicines of all . . . love, prayer, and relationship.

I was not able to be at this gathering in person because I was in Kaua'i; however, I was able to be there in another way . . . in the way that I know best. I wrote her a story and called it "Deer Sister."[8] I sent it to Carl and asked if he would read it at an appropriate time during the meeting, and I would also read it on a sacred mountain in Kaua'i during the same night.

The story is about a deer named Little Flower who always wondered why the moon was white. As she searched and searched for an answer to her question, she came upon a large white feather and knew it belonged to her relative, White Eagle Mother. "Hmmm," she

171

thought to herself, "if I keep this feather, perhaps, I, too, will have some of White Eagle Mother's power to see in many directions. Perhaps one day I will find out about the moon."

Little Flower tucked the feather within her soft brown fur coat and continued on her journey. After a very long time, Little Flower grew tired and fell asleep. Suddenly she was awakened by a familiar smell which meant danger . . . smoke. When she saw the fire raging out of control, her heart felt a big fear. She had no place to run and she felt helpless.

As Little Flower frantically searched for a way to escape, the feather she had found earlier loosened from her coat and fell to the ground. Little Flower picked it up with her mouth and as she did so, she found herself lifting higher and higher off of the ground until she was above the forest . . . above the fire.

As Little Flower flew higher and higher, something strange began to happen. She realized that the great white feather was not in her mouth anymore. Little Flower wondered to herself, "How can I be flying without the feather? I am a deer, and deer cannot fly."

Just then White Eagle Mother came to her and thanked her for bringing her feather back. She told Little Flower that she dropped it while she was flying and that it was Little Flower whom she blessed to bring it back to her. Great White Eagle Mother continued talking to Little Flower and told her that "Each of my feathers holds a prayer for all relatives of Earth. The prayer would have been lost forever, but it was you who found it. However, you in your deer form had no way of bringing it to me in my world, except through the Great Flight of changing forms. You had to cross the bridge from your world into mine . . . and I thank you. You are not just a deer anymore, but you, too, have become a great White Eagle Mother who will carry the prayers of all relatives within the feathers of your wings."

Then Eagle Mother told Little Flower the answer to her long,

172

sought-after question about the moon. She told her that the moon is white because it is the time when all the White Eagle Mothers and Grandmothers show their faces in a great sacred council . . . "And, Little Flower, you are now one of the great White Eagle Mothers whose face will always be seen in the glow of the moon, and your heart's song will be carried with the breath of the wind."

The parallel between my story, which had never been told outside of the prayer ceremony some six months earlier, and Patricia's story was clearly recognized by the workshop participants. It also turns out that Patricia is Catholic and that her Patron Saint is Saint Teresa, known as the "Little Flower." In addition, the date of Susana's death is also Patricia's birthday.

As I choked back tears, I ended the session by telling the group that during a phone call just before Susana died, she told me that she would send me a postcard when she got to the other side. I turned to Patricia and said, "Thank you for the postcard."

Two Hearts

"The Spirit sings through the voice of the heart."
—Joyce C. Mills, Ph.D.[8a]

I learned that postcards can come in many forms. Every February for close to ten years after I lost my twin boys, I found myself in a veil of sadness over the loss. It wasn't a planned time to grieve, it just happened. While I was having a manicure, around the ten year anniversary of their loss, the conversation turned to astrology. At this time, I wasn't really interested in astrology past reading my horoscope in the newspaper for fun. A woman sitting next to me asked, "What sign is your son, Casey?" I thought for a minute, and answered, "Taurus, I think. His birthday is May 27." Quickly she answered, "Nooo, that's not Taurus, that's Gemini. You know, Gemini the twins." A funny feeling whirled though my body when she said that, but I just filed it away in my mind and didn't give it much conscious thought the rest of the day.

A few days later it was Valentine's Day and I was sitting on my bed when nine-year-old Casey energetically bounded into the room and handed me a Valentine he had made for me. The front of the red construction paper card had the typical white doily pasted onto a large red cut-out heart. Smiling, I opened the card and was struck suddenly with astonishment. There in the card were two hearts, one closer to the top of the card and one closer to the bottom of the card, and in the middle the word "twins" was written. I was dumbstruck. This was not the typical message a child writes on a Valentine's card to his mother. With an innocent, inquiring tone I asked, "Casey, this is such a wonderful card. And this word 'twins' . . . could you tell Mommy more about it?" "Sure," he quickly responded. "You know Mom, like there's two of me. There's the warm heart who likes to snuggle really close, and then there's the colder heart who likes to be by himself sometimes." Then looking right into my eyes, he gently repeated, "You know Mom, like there's two of me." I held my precious son very close and said, "Yes, Casey, I know . . . like there is two of you."

This message can be interpreted in many ways. For me, the interpretation was not and is not important. The comfort came through the message. The souls of my twins were all right. I never mourned again.

Steppingstone Fifteen

CHANGING WOMAN TEACHINGS

*"People usually consider walking on water or in thin air a miracle.
But I think the real miracle is not to walk either on water or in thin air,
but to walk on earth."*

—Thich Nhat Hanh[9]

Rebirth and healing can be experienced in relation to each daily occurrence. The sun coming up can be connected to your rebirth into a new day . . . beginning anew. The sun going down can represent a cleansing of worries or concerns. After Hurricane Iniki struck, a Navajo spiritual leader I call Brother told me a story that best describes these concepts. I was on the phone with Thomas, telling him about how I often felt tired and worn out. How I had been having difficulty sleeping peacefully because of the worries that weighed heavily on my mind. He remained silent as he listened, and then just when I thought he was bored to tears with my ramblings, Thomas said, "Sister, do you know about Changing Woman?" Since

I realized that he was about to tell me a wonderful story, he had my undivided attention. "No," I replied, "but I would sure like to know about her."

> *Changing Woman, our eldest Grandmother, is born each day when the sun rises in the east. It is important at that time to turn towards this direction and greet the new day with appreciation . . . perhaps with a prayer saying, "Thank you, Creator, for allowing me to see this new day once again," or with a motion such as raising your hands and touching your heart. During the day, Changing Woman goes through the various stages of life—puberty, middle age, and old age—and finally she travels with the sun as it sets. Face the west direction at this time, pause, and think about any troubles you want to release. Because she is an ancient Grandmother, she has the ability to heal and bless all of her grandchildren. She will take your worries with her so that you can sleep real good, and when you wake up in the morning there is a new day waiting for you.*

After Thomas told me this story, I felt a sense of peacefulness. It was as if Thomas had given me a spiritual prescription for releasing my worries.

Following the teachings woven within this story, take time each day to turn towards the east direction in the morning, stretch your hands, with palms open, above your head, and bring them down placing the palms of your hands over your heart. Take a nice slow, deep breath in through your nose and exhale through your mouth. You are bringing the blessings of the new day to yourself.

Do the same at noontime and during late-afternoon. Finally, face west as the sun is about to set, take a slow, deep breath, and visualize all of your worries flowing into an imaginery basket. Once the basket is full, imagine handing it to Changing Woman. It doesn't matter if you are in the city or in the country. Nor does it matter what time of year it is. What matters is that you allow the blessings of Changing Woman to touch your heart with a sense of healing and inner peace.

CHAPTER SIXTEEN

The Cigar Man

"An angel has wings and lives up in the sky.
They talk to children in their hearts."

—Anonymous, Age 6[10]

*I*t was getting towards evening on December 31, 1995, when my husband, Eddie, and I decided to swing by the lushly flowered Hyatt Hotel and drop off holiday gifts for some of our friends who were working there. We were both very tired and decided to spend New Year's Eve alone. No great social plans or hoopla, just a quiet evening of being together.

After we had dropped off the gifts, we agreed that it would be a wonderful treat to sip a tall guava drink on the inviting, open-air terrace while watching the magical Kaua'i sunset. We immediately noticed two empty chairs near the music area and decided that it would be a perfect spot for us to enjoy both the spectacular ocean view and the happy sounds of our local musicians. However, just as we were settling into our chairs, our romantic rapture was quickly cut short by the overwhelmingly pungent and enormously offensive smell of a large cigar. Our response was, "Just what we need . . . someone smelling up our beautiful Kaua'i air . . . YUK!"

We pondered the idea of leaving the hotel entirely or moving to another spot. As we glancing around, we noticed an empty table far enough away to avoid the oppressive smell, so we decided to stay. Next to us were a couple, smiling and taking pictures of each other. The man had a delightfully warm presence about him. His large frame and white hair reminded me of a gentle white bear. The woman was equally lovely, with short dark hair, a soft smile, and soulful eyes. Just as I was thinking to myself, "I'll ask if they want us to take a picture of them together," they turned to us and asked us that very question. When Eddie got up to photograph them, the man noticed he was wearing a large gold angel pin on his sweatshirt. "Where did you get that angel?" the man asked. "It's really wonderful." We told him that we had a shop that sells angels of all kinds, and immediately the man and woman responded enthusiastically by telling us that they knew the store and were there last year when we first opened. They reminisced about the good feelings they had had there.

At this point Eddie and I introduced ourselves by name and they did the same. We were enjoying our meeting so much that we asked John and Jeraldene to join us at our table. Our conversation and friendship blossomed from there.

They asked about how the shop came to be. I said that it was kind of a long story, but John and Jeraldene said that they had plenty of time and really wanted to know. I related that while I was in Oregon, I had been writing a chapter for a new book I had been working on, when I began to become aware of the feeling that angels were nearby. I mentioned that I had never thought of angels before in any particular way . . . I liked them, to be sure, but that was about it. As I was writing this chapter on humorous and inspirational encounters people had just prior to their deaths, I felt the presence of my friend's brother, who had died the year before of AIDS. What was strange was that I never met him in person, but for some reason I couldn't get him out of my mind.

I felt compelled to call my friend, Charlee, who lived in New Jersey, and tell her of my feelings about her brother, Gershon, and the angels. She told me that this was around the anniversary of his death and asked if I had seen the memorial she had written about him. When I said that I hadn't, Charlee said that she would fax it to me immediately and that I would understand why I kept feeling that angels were around. While holding the fax in my hands, my eyes immediately focused on the last line, which was one of Gershon's favorite quotes from Shakespeare. In large bold letters it read, "Goodnight, Sweet Prince, Flights of Angels Sing Thee to Thy Rest." Quickly, I called Charlee back and we spent over an hour just talking about Gershon and the angels.

That same evening, after going to dinner with a colleague and friend, we found ourselves wandering in a wonderful angel store in Oregon called Angels and Us. For some reason I began buying angels of all kinds . . . angel cards, angel statues, angel wrapping paper, angel incense, angel pins, angel dolls, and on and on. What was really bizarre was that I had no idea why, or to whom, all these would be given as gifts. I only knew that I had to have the ones that seemed to speak to me the most.

Jeraldene and John were exchanging smiles and twinkling glances all the while I spoke. I went on to tell them that the next day, when I shared this story with a good friend, Sister Katherine Knoll, over a delightful Oregon home-style breakfast, I had a true vision of an angel store in the town of Hanapepe on the west side of Kaua'i. The sumptuous breakfast was literally blocked out by my vision of this store. At the time, Eddie was working as a bartender while exploring other possible avenues of work on Kaua'i. Suddenly I blurted out, "Katherine, please don't think I'm nuts, but I know what we are supposed to do. It's an all-angel store!" I then proceeded to describe the vision in detail. The more I described, the more effervescent I felt.

In her inimitable deep voice, Katherine said, "So what are you waiting for, girl, call Eddie and tell him." After gobbling down a few bites, we left most of our breakfast sitting there and rushed back to Katherine's office and I called Eddie. What was most unusual was that Eddie's normal it's-not-going-to-work type of skepticism was absent. His immediate response was "Let's do it!" And so "Uncle Eddie's Aloha Angels" was born.

Jeraldene and John listened with great absorption. As they glanced back and forth to each other, John asked Jeraldene to share why they were here in Kaua'i this time. She agreed, and this time Eddie and I were the receivers of their special story. On January 5, 1995, one year earlier, their eighteen-year-old son had died of a heart attack. He had been in excellent health, an athlete with a wonderful future ahead of him, when suddenly, without warning, his heart gave out and he died. Jeraldene said that they were here to honor this first anniversary of his passing with a ceremony. Both she and John said that they felt the presence of the angels the entire time they were in Kaua'i and that truly the angels had brought us together. Eddie and I even thought that the man smoking the obnoxious cigar was an angel in disguise, orchestrating our meeting! John and Jeraldene agreed, because they too had smelled the smoke and moved because of it. "Perhaps we should send him a thank-you note," Eddie quipped. We all laughed in agreement.

As the conversation unfolded, John shared that he had met Jeraldene in a group many years ago while doing grief work after losing his precious daughter, Alexia, when she was eight years old. What led Jeraldene into this work was another loss she had experienced: her first son, Sean, had died when he, too, was eight years old. Both Eddie and I sat in awe and wonder at the courage of these two special people as they shared these tragic experiences with us as lovingly as one gives the most sacred of gifts from the heart. The conversation continued as the sun dropped its glowing light into the Kaua'i ocean before us. The night sky was just beginning to display its island magnificence as luminescent colors of pinks, lavenders, and yellows emerged upwards.

Somehow, time was suspended as we continued to share all aspects of our lives, personal, professional, and spiritual. John and Jeraldene noticed one of the many necklaces I was wearing—a silver dreamcatcher and a buffalo-bone feather hanging from a simple thin silver chain. When they asked about it, we shared some of our experiences with our Native American relatives and how we had come to believe that we are all relatives in life. Jeraldene and John also talked about their experiences with Native peoples and how much their lives had been enriched by these teachings.

At this point, the conversation returned to the memorial ceremony for their son Alex. I asked Jeraldene if she knew where she wanted to have it. She replied that she wasn't quite sure as yet but felt a place would reveal itself. As Jeraldene continued talking, a special beach on the west side of Kaua'i called Polihale came to mind. I explained that it was called the "jumping off place of the spirits" by many people over here. Jeraldene's eyes lit up and said that friends here had told them about that beach, but they hadn't been there yet. After a few moments of reflective silence, Jeraldene said that she felt it was the right place for the ceremony. She then paused and looked at John, then back at us, and asked if we would help them with the ceremony. I glanced at Eddie and without hesitation agreed to participate in any way possible. We talked about what was important for them in expressing their honor for the spirit of Alex.

Jeraldene said that she and John had been given a drum and many sacred herbs, such as tobacco, sage, and cedar, but had left all their things back in Utah. As it was, Eddie and I had all of what she wanted to use for the ceremony and were honored to be able to share what we had with them. Jeraldene also wanted to prepare a basket of fruit and place it in the ocean as a gift for the spirit of her son. We chose the time of day to have the ceremony—sunset . . . a time of rest and peacefulness. Each aspect of the memorial for Alex unfolded naturally, with a feeling of a gentle, light spirit guiding its direction. Perhaps the ceremony was being sculpted by the loving wings of the angels.

The fourth of January arrived with the gentle mist of a warm Kaua'i rain. John, Jeraldene, two of their friends, their two young daughters, and Eddie and myself met at the beach. We spread out a large blanket on which each of us placed the special offerings we had brought. We sang songs, told stories, passed photographs, shared the offerings we brought, and said prayers in honor of beloved Alex.

When the glowing sun was descending into the ocean's azure horizon, Jeraldene took the basket filled with all of Alex's favorite fruit and passed it to each one of us. We then placed an offering of private meaning in it for Alex's safe journey to the spirit world. When the basket had made its way full circle, we all watched as Jeraldene and John walked slowly towards the ocean with basket in hand. Some private prayers were said by all and then Jeraldene knelt down and gently placed her offering on the powder-like white sand, just as the waves lapped onto the shore's edge. We stood silently and watched as the waves grew stronger . . . as if reaching towards the gift that was being presented. John had wandered off down the long, white soft-sanded beach, all the while drumming on a large hand-held drum that had been made for me by someone I call my sister, Jill Hagen. Half Jewish and half Onondaga, Jill's only daughter, Terry, was one of the very brave firefighters who had been killed the year before while fighting a devastating fire in Colorado. She made this drum for me shortly after her loss. Lovingly hand-painted with many symbols, Jill sent the drum to me with the hope I would use it for healing. When John asked if he could use one of my drums, I showed him the three that I had brought with me. Without hesitation, he chose the one Jill had made. Perhaps he recognized the heartbeat of a daughter-angel far away.

When the basket eventually disappeared into the ocean's embrace, we shared the sumptuous food prepared by the friends of John and Jeraldene. With laughter and a sense of gratefulness, we remembered the big brawny man with the pungent cigar and how the tapestry of a new friendship is woven together by the invisible wings of the angels.

Steppingstone Sixteen

*"All of life can become ritual. When it does,
our experience of life changes radically and the ordinary
becomes consecrated."*

—Rachel Naomi Remen, M.D.[11]

*E*ach of us will have a different purpose for wanting to create a ritual or a ceremony in our lives. Jeraldene and John wanted a ceremony honoring the life of their son, Alex. A couple I worked with decided to renew their relationship after separating and bought a fruit tree for their yard. They planted it just as the sun was coming up, a time of day that symbolized new beginnings. They agreed to water it together and make sure it grew healthy and strong. The fruit grown was symbolic of the fruits gained from the love they shared.

Another example is that of Mary, a forty-two-year-old woman who created a ritual for honoring the death of an unborn baby girl she had miscarried when she was in her early twenties. Because the baby was only carried to the first trimester, the spiritual and emo-

185

tional need for a time of mourning went unrecognized by her family and doctor. For years she wondered about this baby and would get tearful around the anniversary date of the loss. As part of her ritual, Mary decided to write a letter to her baby and tell her about the love she carried in her heart for her, as well as about herself and her family. She decided to go to a special place by the ocean and read the letter to the baby just as the sun was setting. She then scooped out a space in the sand, placed the letter with pictures of herself, her husband, and her family in the hole and burned them, along with a handful of dried leaves from her garden. When all was ash, Mary covered the burnt offerings with sand and placed white daisies on her baby's grave site. With tears flowing freely, Mary finished telling me her story by saying, "I now know my Daisy is with God."

To honor the first birthday of my Goddaughter, Sophia Ming Lu, who was adopted from an orphanage in China, we gathered with family and friends and created a ceremony different from the usual cake and ice cream party. We began with a talking circle, in which each of us shared our hopes, wishes, and prayers for Sophia's life. Some participants told stories from their own lives, some sang songs, and some read poetry.

One of Sophia's adopted Aunties is a basket weaver. Auntie Laura brought along a special, but unfinished basket for Sophia and passed it to each of us in the circle to add our personal weaving touch. The finished product became a "Blessing Basket" for Sophia to keep for all time. Each strand of the straw-like material was woven with a special prayer by each person participating in this basket-weaving ceremony. We presented the basket to Sophia's mother, Aimee, and asked her to find a special place for it in their home. As Sophia grows, she will most likely encounter challenges as we all do, but perhaps the blessings woven within the basket will help to remind her of the love and support she was given when she was very small.

✻   ✻   ✻

Although these stories are different, they are united by a common theme: *we need to be active participants in our healings and in our celebrations.* No one knows our personal stories or healing needs better than we do, and I believe that deep within the recesses of our heart, we yearn to tell our stories in many forms so that we can heal. Rituals and ceremonies can help us.

You are invited to use the following outline to help identify what *your* purpose is for creating a ritual or ceremony in your life. Ask yourself, "What do I need right now in order to reconnect to my life's magic? Is it to

- Build inner strength?
- Reaffirm individual identity?
- Acknowledge a rite of passage? (Birth, puberty, graduation, marriage, menopause, grandparenthood, death.)
- Reaffirm a sense of connectedness with my family . . . community . . . the world?
- Reaffirm a sense of connectedness with nature . . . animals . . . plants . . . weather elements . . . cycles of the day, and so on?
- Restore balance and harmony within myself, my relationship, my family?
- Acknowledge, honor, and celebrate a life accomplishment?
- To release pain, fear, struggle?
- Reaffirm a sense of relationship with the sacred?
- Provide a safe arena in which the process of healing can take place?

Feel free to add any purpose for a ritual or ceremony not mentioned on this list.

Creating Your Own Ritual or Ceremony

Now that you have identified your purpose for needing a ritual or ceremony in your life, it is time to *create* one. The worksheet on page 190 was designed to help you formulate your ideas.

Take time to explore what you need in your life right now. If you wish, you can use this framework with your family, friends, or business associates. When trying to solve our problems, we often need to expand our vision so that we can see with the eyes of the eagle rather than with the narrow vision of the mouse. Rituals and ceremonies can help us to do just that.

WORKSHEET FOR CREATING A RITUAL OR CEREMONY

1. What is the purpose of this ritual/ceremony? (Use the outline provided on p. 187 to determine this.)
2. What materials will I need to create this ritual/ceremony? (The couple who renewed their relationship used a fruit tree, a shovel, and water. Mary wrote a letter, brought pictures, leaves, and flowers.)
3. Do I want anyone present to help me with this ritual/ceremony? (Remember Jaimi and her Bowl of Light? I was present as she emptied her stones.) If so, with whom do I want to share this experience?
4. Where will this ritual/ceremony take place?
5. When will it take place—time of day, what date?
6. What will I need to celebrate the closure of this ritual/ceremony? (For example, foods, gifts, and so on.)

A story that best ends this steppingstone is one shared by the tea master, Shoshitsu Sen XV. In his book *Tea Life and Tea Mind,* he tells a story of a tea grower who invited a most respected tea master, Rikyu, to have tea. Overcome with the excitement of Rikyu's acceptance, the tea grower's "hand trembled and he performed badly, dropping the tea scoop and knocking the tea whisk over." While the other guests and disciples of Rikyu snickered, the tea master Rikyu was visibly moved to say, "It was the finest."

It seems that on the way home, one of the disciples asked Rikyu why he was so impressed with "such a shameful performance." In his great wisdom, Rikyu answered, "This man did not invite me with the idea of showing off his skill. He simply wanted to serve me tea with his whole heart. He devoted himself completely to making a bowl of tea for me, not worrying about errors. I was struck by that sincerity."

This wise teaching as shared by the Japanese tea master, Shoshitsu Sen XV, reminds us that the most important rule to remember in any ritual is to serve with "the sincere heart of the host."

Worksheet for Ritual

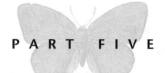

PART FIVE

Giveaway. . . Sharing the Vision

". . . . When you come on something good, first thing to do is share it with whomever you can find; that way, the good spreads out where no telling it will go."

—Forrest Carter[1]

Many religions and cultures embrace the philosophy of giveaway in one form or another, helping us to understand that we are not the owners of things but are simply the caretakers. We are merely the keepers of the stories, objects, or lessons entrusted to us—and the time will come when we will have to pass on whatever we have learned or been given. Like an old family quilt that is passed on from generation to generation, the relational message of passing on whatever we have learned or been given becomes the sacred heirloom that not only enriches our lives, but also enriches the lives of those to whom it is given. It becomes the legacy on which we build individual acquisitions into community endeavors, and it is the landscape on which both the inner and outer ecology of life thrive.

CHAPTER SEVENTEEN

The Sacred Pipe

*"How wonderful it is
that nobody need wait a single moment
before starting to improve the world."*

—Anne Frank[2]

efore Susana died, I spent many weekends with her. On one such weekend in August 1988, prior to her surgery, I thought we would be able to go on a camping trip with others who had participated in our Turtle Island retreats. Carl Hammerschlag had organized the trip in the hope of bringing us together to talk about our visions for future retreats. Since Susana realized she was too weak to go, she decided to stay home. However, she insisted I go with the others and that she would be just fine. The night before I left, Susana wanted to have a Giveaway Ceremony. I had never heard of this ceremony, since I was very new to Native American teachings.

Susana asked my friend Rita and me to sit in a circle with her. Susana proceeded to light some sage and cedar, which she thoughtfully placed in a large abalone shell. On an old Navajo blanket she carefully placed many objects before us which were sacred to her, such as a hand-beaded leather pouch, a tiger's eye stone, an amber necklace, a Pipe with white feathers, and a small rose quartz turtle. Susana told us that since she had been ill, many things that belonged to her were *asking* to be given away. She explained that in the Native American tradition we are not the owners of things; instead we are the keepers and that a time would come to give them away to other people. As Susana picked up each item, she told how she had gotten it and then gave it either to Rita or to me. After a short time, Susana picked up the Pipe with a white stone bowl and four white feathers hanging from its stem. The Pipe had been used by Willie Whitefeather, a Cherokee medicine man living in Arizona. He worked primarily with children and had used this pipe with them in his teachings and prayers. After the summer he had given it to Susana. She said that the Pipe had been *talking* to her, telling her that it was time to give it away. As Susana handed me the Pipe, she said that it was to be given "to her sister of spirit who works with children." At this time, I did not know the depth of teachings that came with the Pipe. I only knew that it was very Sacred and that I was open to learning.

The next morning we all got up early and together prepared for our campout. Susana was delighted we were still going and packed whatever she could for us. Rita and I were picked up by Steven, a young man we had never met. We piled into the front seat of his truck and off we went. I promised Susana a blow-by-blow account of our trip.

The truck bounced along the dusty Arizona roads as we shared stories of our lives. By the time we reached our destination of Prescott, we felt as if we had known each other for many lifetimes. I am sure that we did. We unloaded all of our camping gear and prepared for the weekend's happenings. It promised to be a time of fun, prayer, song, creativity, hiking, and rest—a beef stew sort of weekend, with a mixture of a little of everything going into the pot.

That evening we gathered around the campfire. I had told Carl about the Pipe and he suggested that I put it by the fire, along with the rattles we had made earlier that day. He said that we were going to have a Talking Circle. There were over twenty of us who gathered in the circle. As an eagle feather was passed to each of us, we shared whatever was on our minds and in our hearts. I talked about receiving the Pipe, acknowledging that I had received a gift of great meaning. When it was time for Carl to speak, he held a hawk feather, with one claw still attached, and said that it had been given to him during a ceremony known as Sun Dance. I vaguely knew what he was referring to because I had read about it in his book *Dancing Healers*.[3] Carl said that he knew it was time to give this feather away. With the evening campfire glowing, Carl came over to me and said that this feather was for me to continue telling the stories. When he handed me the feather, a strange feeling I still cannot explain came over me. I brushed it on my face and along my arms. I smelled it and even held it close to my ears, as if listening to its message.

Later that evening I asked Carl about the feather. He said to have patience and it, like the Pipe, would lead me in the right direction. By the time morning came, I realized that I had to go to a Sun Dance ceremony . . . I didn't know how I would get there or even where one was going to be held, or even if I, as a white person, could go. What I did know is that I had to find out. And so the giveaway of the Pipe and the feather had opened a doorway for new learnings.

As the months passed, I learned that the Sun Dance is one of the most sacred of ceremonies celebrated by the Plains Indian people, given to them by White Buffalo Calf Woman as one of the seven sacred teachings of the Pipe. At the time of the Sun Dance ceremony, a great tree is brought to the center of an arbor. From the time it is cut, it is carried without touching the ground until it is uprighted by the people. Many tobacco ties are made by each person offering prayers, which are fastened to this tree. These small bundles are made by placing sacred tobacco in the center of each square of cloth of varying colors—red, yellow, black, white, blue, and green—and each bundle is joined together with red yarn and then fastened to the great sacred Sun Dance tree.

This ceremony is four days of intense prayer . . . of focused prayer. Dancers commit themselves through mind, body, and spirit to dance in the blazing sun, offering the one thing they have come into this world with . . . their flesh. The men pierce their flesh by lying on a buffalo hide and allowing a medicine man to grip their skin above the pectoral muscle and pierce a sliver of bone through it. They each tie a long rope around the sacred tree and it is to this rope that they fasten themselves from the bone pierced through their chests. And then they dance for the blessings of all peoples. When they feel that the time is right within their souls, the men pull back from the tree until the flesh is torn from their bodies as an offering to the Great Spirit and as a total commitment to the sacred pathways they follow.

As part of this sacred ceremony, women dance as well. They do not have to pierce their skin, because they give of their blood each month and they give of their bodies in birth. Yet the commitment is the same. They dance for four days just like the men, boys, and old men, fasting the whole time, no food and no water, beginning and ending each day of dancing in a sweat lodge.

Each dancer carries a Sacred Pipe. During certain times a dancer will choose someone who is on the outside of the arbor circle and offer his or her Pipe. The person who is offered the Pipe shares it with whoever wishes to join the circle. It was during one of these times that I received a great teaching again.

A Pipe was given to a Native American woman standing near me. She began to form her circle and I, as always, went to join in and pray. She looked up at me and pointedly asked, "Are you Indian?" "No," I replied with gulping hesitancy. "Well, you can't sit with us; this is just for Indians." Her distasteful glare and straight-shooting words left me feeling as if my heart had been pierced by a misguided arrow. Of course, I understood that she harbored deep-seated pain and anger towards white people for their continued abuse of her people along with assaults on their land, and she probably saw me as just another white person coming in to exploit their sacred ways. I could not try to explain that I related to her pain as a Jewish woman whose people had also endured human atrocities of enormous magnitude. I also could not explain to her how much these sacred ceremonies meant to me, nor about the many Native American people with whom I had developed deep-hearted relationships, and how committed I felt to the teachings. I knew that I would just sound like another wanna-be from California. So I simply nodded my head indicating that I understood; I turned and walked away.

Tears welled up in my eyes as I blindly walked back through an opening in the fields, past the Sun Dance camp where the tipis stood and past the many sweat lodges. No one was around in this open field. Through my tears, though, I saw someone coming towards me. As he got closer, I saw it was George, a man who is known as a dreamspeaker. His hair was long, salt-and-pepper colored and blowing wispily in the warm breezes of the day. I had met George the first night of the Sun Dance during a children's sweat lodge ceremony.

"Hey there," George said to me. "How you doing?" Sobbing, sniffing, and somewhat choking, I responded by saying, "Not so good, George." Concerned, he asked, "What's goin' on with you?" I repeated the story of the Pipe, the woman, and her words to me. I told him maybe it was a sign I didn't belong here . . . being white and all.

George moved closer and looked directly into my eyes. With a deep, resonant voice he said, "Why are you giving her your power?" He repeated the question again with even greater strength in his voice, "Why are you giving her your power? I know you know better than that. We used your Pipe in a sweat with the children. It was the Creator that brought you here. Not a person." I stood completely still, riveted to his words.

George continued. "What I want you to do is go into a sweat lodge and pray for her. If she said that to you during this time of Sun Dance, then she doesn't know the real meaning of the Pipe. Pray for her." Then George held his hand up and made a motion as if screwing a lightbulb into an invisible socket. Giving a slight but definite twist to his wrist, he said, "Sister, turn it around . . . pray. Sometime during this Sun Dance you, too, will be offered a Pipe. Find this woman and offer it to her. Unity, love, peace are the teachings of the Pipe. Not prejudice. You heard what Martin Highbear said as our Intercessor of this Sun Dance; he began this ceremony with the words, 'Leave all prejudice outside . . . bringing it in will only hurt the dancers . . . it will make them sick'. "

And so, I did as George asked. I went into a woman's sweat lodge and prayed for her. The next day I was offered a Pipe just as George predicted. I went in search of the woman, found her, offered the Pipe to her, and asked if she would like to join us. "NO!" she snapped back at me; then she turned and walked away. I had to see that, too. It was part of the teachings. I learned once again that prayer is not about trying to get what we want from others but about healing our own hearts and reestablishing our relationship to something greater than ourselves.

Over the last decade of participating in many ceremonies, as well as living and working with Native people, I have learned that these experiences are not to be romanticized or collected like charms on a bracelet to be shown off. When I first thought about writing this story, I questioned if I even had the right to do so as a white person. I spoke about it with many of my Native American relatives, including Martin Highbear at the Sun Dance. He pointed to the arbor and to the sacred tree and said, "Joyce, see that tree? Do you see the colors of those prayers? . . . Black, white, red, and yellow. All of the colors of the Creator's children. And blue for Grandfather Sky and green for our Mother Earth. It was prophesied that when all of the colors dance together in the Great Arbor, there will be peace in our world. This was prophesied by the Medicine people. You are a child of color. You are a storyteller. Go and pray with your Pipe. Take care of it and it will take care of you." And so I did. . . . And so I do.

Martin Highbear died on September 2, 1995. His gifts continue to be given away through the stories he shared with many.

Note: The word "Pipe" was capitalized throughout, to acknowledge its sacredness to the Native American people.

Steppingstone Seventeen

*"If we have no peace, it is because we have forgotten
that we belong to each other."*

—Mother Teresa[4]

*I*n the field of ecology the term *global warming* brings with it an ominous warning that our planet is in serious danger. I think our planet *is* in serious danger, not only from the perspective of outer-ecological threats, but also from the equally important inner-ecological threats, such as those relating to cuts in vital educational and health-care programs. I believe our missions as human beings in this upcoming twenty-first century is to promote *global caring* . . . a different kind of global warming. One way that all of us can participate in this goal is through rituals and ceremonies. Caring will ultimately lead to healing.

Several years ago, I received a letter from Barbara Omaha, a spiritual sister from the Ojibway tribe, a Pipe carrier, and a Sun Dancer, telling me that June 21, 1996, was designated as a day of prayer and ceremony for world peace. The request for this special day of Global Healing came from Arvol Looking Horse, 19th Generation Keeper of the Sacred White Buffalo Calf Pipe for the Lakota, Dakota, and Nakota Nations.[5] I end this chapter with his word-for-word declaration in its entirety. It is my hope that Arvol Looking Horse's plea for world peace and harmony be the wings on which Global Healing takes flight and soars, and that the spiritual message of June 21 be a day that is celebrated every day of every year.

> *I, Arvol Looking Horse, 19th Generation Keeper of the Sacred White Buffalo Calf Pipe for the Lakota, Dakota, and Nakota Nations ask that all Nations upon Mother Earth declare June 21, 1996 World Peace and Prayer Day. According to spiritual leaders and Elders who gathered at the United Nations to present their prophecies—and again at Six Nations, Canada—the "signs" of Indigenous peoples' prophecies have shown themselves. The prophecies tell us it is time to begin mending the Sacred Hoop and begin global healing by working towards world peace and harmony.*
>
> *The birth of the White Buffalo Calf lets us know we are at a crossroads—either return to balance or face global disaster. It is our duty to return back to the sacred places and pray for world peace—if we do not do this our children will suffer.*
>
> *At Grey Horn Butte, before the White Buffalo Woman brought the Sacred Pipe to our ancestors, a Seer was traveling in the Sacred Black Hills—Paha Sapa, "heart of everything that is." The Seer came upon a large tipi. When he went in the tipi, he saw the Sacred Pipe in the North and the Sacred Bundle of Bows and Arrows in the South. According to the Star Knowledge there are six stars which designated six sacred sites*

within the Black Hills—these places are sacred places to pray. We are told there is a sacred place every hundred miles around Mother Earth. We ask all people to return to these places and pray from their hearts with us. The ceremony begins 10 A.M. South Dakota (Mountain) time.

It has been decided, according to the Star Knowledge, that June 21st is the time to pray. Indigenous people of Turtle Island will begin their spiritual journey on horseback from Wahpeton, Saskatchewan, Canada to Grey Horn Butte (known as Devils Tower) in the Black Hills of Wyoming. There, Indigenous peoples will pray with the Sacred Bundle Keepers to begin the restoration of peace and balance. We ask all Peoples to begin organizing their ceremonies at their sacred sites or in the manner in which they pray so that they will be praying at the same time as we are from their own spiritual center.

So far, we have spoken to leaders from around the world and each has committed to work towards supporting June 21st, 1996. We ask all people of all faiths to respond and support our efforts towards world peace and harmony—our circle of life where there is no ending and no beginning. May peace be with you all.

—19th Generation Keeper of the Sacred White Buffalo
　Calf Pipe

Arvol Looking Horse

CHAPTER EIGHTEEN

The Mystery of Life

*"Everything in life is a story. . . . It provides us
with the sense of living mystery in life."*

—Laurens van der Post[6]

While attending the 1996 National Speakers Conference in Orlando, Florida, we were treated to a keynote presentation by Arun Gandhi,[7] the grandson of *the* Mahatma Gandhi. Mr. Gandhi told many stories related to his grandfather's beliefs in nonviolence, but one in particular stayed with me throughout the five days of the conference. For me, this story encapsulated the core soul message of Giveaway. I share this story with you in the way that I remember it.

> *Many centuries ago there was a great king who wanted to know about the mysteries of life. He went to the home of a sage and beseeched him to tell him the mystery. The sage went into the back room and came out with a single grain of wheat. He handed the grain of wheat to the king without saying a word. The king thought he was making fun of him and, in a huff, he took the grain of wheat, walked out, and went back to his palace.*
>
> *The king was confused and didn't know what to do with the grain of wheat. Was it the mystery of life—or wasn't it? Not sure of what he really had, but at the same time quite sure that he had something not to be discarded, he had a special gold box made, into which he put the grain of wheat. Every few days the king looked at the grain of wheat in the box, but nothing was happening. The king was feeling very frustrated, annoyed, and disappointed until one day he came upon a wise Indian person who explained everything that had taken place with the grain of wheat and the box. The king then asked the wise person to please tell him what is the mystery of life. Once again the great king was told that "That is the mystery of life." The Indian wise person continued, "Unless that grain of wheat is put in its environment so that it comes in touch with all the different elements of its life, it cannot grow, it cannot produce . . . it will do nothing. If you keep it in this box, it will be a dead grain of wheat, nothing will happen to it."*

Arun Gandhi said that this was the philosophy of his grandfather in relation to life and nonviolence: if we take the teachings and philosophies we learn and put them away in books, only reading them occasionally, they become somewhat meaningless. But if we take them out and use them in our daily lives, these *grains of wheat* will have the opportunity to grow and flourish.

Later that evening and all through the conference, I found myself thinking about the gift of this story. Clearly, it was not a step-by-step model for overcoming fear and violence in our world, nor was it a didactic approach for catapulting our careers as speakers or marketing wizards. For me, the story carried a deeper message ribboned with wisdom. I believe that just as the sage had placed a grain of wheat in the king's hand, so too did Gandhi give each of us in the audience a grain of wheat by sharing the story . . . he put the mystery of life within our grasp. It is up to us to choose what we do with it: we can nurture the grain so that our lives blossom with meaning and sustenance, or we could place it in a box, as did the king, and continue to search for something more—on one hand, knowing that we were given something special, yet on the other hand, never feeling satisfied with the gifts we have been given.

Many times in life we search and search for the mysteries that life has to offer. We want more, bigger, better, faster, and so on, but these material things keep us from experiencing the true mysteries and miracles of life. What are those mysteries and miracles? I am truly not wise enough to answer such a question, but I know that for each of us they will be different. I ponder the beauty of a sunset, the glow of a full moon, the feeling of a gentle rain caressing my skin in the midst of a warm summer day, or the sound of the deep-bellied giggle of a little child.

On that warm Florida evening in the grand ballroom of the Marriott Hotel, a grain of wheat was placed in my hands. How will I nurture it? Where will I plant it? I am not quite sure. Perhaps it is already planted, as the story continues to be told.

Steppingstone Eighteen

PLANTING THE SEEDS, REAPING THE HARVEST

"Plant Seeds. Plant thoughts. Plant yourself. Care for yourself in a way that will produce the healthiest, most beautiful plants. Don't forget that one of the plants in the garden you are tending is you."

—Bernie Siegel, M.D.[8]

Before my Bubbie died, she gave me a white, square shawl she had crocheted many years earlier. With delicate designs crocheted into it and a thick border of fringes, this shawl is one of my most treasured gifts. I take it with me to all my workshops and share the stories of my grandmother through its spirit. Oftentimes, during or after a workshop, people tell me stories of their own grandparents. Stories they remembered after seeing the shawl. I know that a time will come when I will give away the shawl to one of my children or grandchildren and the stories will continue.

The sad part is that I know very few stories about my grandmother's life. When she came to this country in the early 1900s from Russia, it was shameful for her to speak in Yiddish in public. She wanted to be

"Americana," as she would say, and she stopped telling the stories of the old country. Now she was in America. I never heard these stories from my mother either. Nothing brought home this fact more than when my precious mother died recently. While looking at family pictures, I realized that I knew very little about my ancestors. Oh, I knew most of their names and whom I am named after, but I know very little about their stories . . . their lives. This leaves a hollow space within the garden of my life and subsequently in the lives of my children. And so I hold the shawl close, as its delicately crocheted stitches provide story seeds lying dormant within the moist earth of my life.

Steppingstone Eighteen is meant to help you reconnect to the magic of the story seeds quietly waiting to be nurtured and awakened within the garden of your own life. The most important thing to remember is that you are already a storyteller. You have been telling stories from the time you were very small. Stories are all around you, but most of all they are in the sacred spaces of your heart. And it is through the heart we see our greatest visions and honor our inner dreams.

Gathering Our Story Seeds

Perhaps you have a piece of jewelry, an article of clothing, a shawl, blanket, fishing pole, a photograph, or some other special object that was given to you by someone special. Find a stretch of quiet time and see what stories you can connect with these objects. Maybe you will recall a favorite holiday gathering, a joyful celebration, or an important life-cycle event. Use the following page or another piece of paper to write down the tiniest shimmer of a memory. These small glints become the seeds from which your stories will grow. As these stories begin to take root and grow, share them as you would share the sweetest of strawberries with a special someone in your life and enjoy reaping the harvest.

Story Seeds

Suggestions for Releasing the Storyteller Within

- Make a list of your hobbies, Interests, talents, or favorite experiences from the present, from when you were a teenager, and from when you were a young child.

- Next, take some quiet time to remember an experience connected to each of them, such as a time you learned one of these hobbies or skills from a grandparent . . . or a time you went hiking, camping, or fishing, and so on. Think about where you were when you learned or experienced them.

- Then find a quiet place, choose one of the experiences, and write about it. Don't worry about grammar, spelling, punctuation, and so on. Just write and have fun.

- After you have written about the experience, find a friend or family member—or use a tape recorder—and just tell your story. You may read it from what you have written or tell it the best way you remember it. Begin your story something like this. . . "and that reminds me of a story. . . ."

Enjoy, discover, and let the storyteller within play. . . . It is just as Gandhi told his grandson: we must take the seed out of the box, plant it, nurture it, and love it . . . that *is* the Mystery of Life.

CHAPTER NINETEEN

Bread of Love

"The soul unfolds itself, like a lotus of countless petals."

—Kahlil Gibran[9]

As a little girl of five, I remember sitting at our yellow Formica table, happily watching my Bubbie mix flour, eggs, yeast, a dash of salt, and water in a large bowl, preparing our Sabbath challah (a sacred bread made especially to celebrate the beginning of the Jewish Sabbath on Friday night). Her delicate hands would take the dough out of the bowl and knead it until it was perfectly smooth. "Joyce-ala, nah," ("Joyce, here") she would say, handing me a piece of dough pulled off her larger piece. This was a moment I eagerly anticipated . . . a piece of dough from my Bubbie. She and I would pound the dough down, put it in the bowl, and repeat this process three times until it had risen sufficiently to braid. We would then smear egg yolk on the braided dough and put it in the oven to bake. The luscious smell of fresh baking bread would swirl through our one-bedroom apartment on Grant Avenue in the Bronx, filling every corner with a feeling of warmth and love.

As I recall those special times with my Bubbie, I am reminded of a story that I first came across in a wonderful book by storyteller Naomi Steinberg entitled *The Dybbuk and Other Stories for Reading Aloud.*[10] The story is called "The Rebbitsin's Challah," which means "The Rabbi's Wife's Challah." Since that time, I have heard the story told in many different ways, but because Naomi tells it best, I share with you the essence of her version. The story in its entirety can be found in her book.

Once, a long time ago, there was a very bright but poor young man who was to marry a very plain and simple daughter of a wealthy merchant. The young man felt very good about this match, because he thought it was the end of his poverty. But that was not to be. A terrible strife swept through the land and the merchant became ill and lost all of his wealth. The only thing the young man could do was to take a job as the town's rabbi.

The young man was very angry at this turn of events. But the young Rebbetsin, the Rabbi's wife, was not bothered by these challenges. She worked hard in her home and planted a vegetable garden in order to help with the much-needed income. It was said that she even found time to clean the synagogue and keep the candlesticks polished. Most importantly, every Friday she would go into town and buy flour and bake her own

Sabbath challah to be shared with their small congregation. Most of the time her loaves would turn out misshapen and sometimes even burned on the bottoms. She was not a very skilled baker.

On Friday night the young rabbi would drone on and on to his congregants, somewhat taken by the sound of his own voice. But, in fact, his words were empty and boring, and most of his congregants were bored and uninspired. Finally, when he finished, he would say the prayer over the wine and unveil the challah. Each time he shuddered at the sight of the misshapen bread and secretly wished he had the money to buy challah from the best baker in town. For him, his wife's challah symbolized his failure.

After saying the Ha-motzi (the prayer over the bread), he would pass pieces of the challah to the congregants. But their experience was quite different from his. Something magical seemed to happen as they ate the Rebbitsin's challah. Their blank, bored eyes began to sparkle with joy and lightness. They happily greeted one another with warm and loving wishes for a "Good Shabbos." Everyone's heart was filled with pleasure . . . everyone's except the Rabbi, because all he could taste was plain bread.

As the weeks and months passed, the synagogue grew full with people from distant villages. The Rabbi continued with his boring sermons, but when the congregants tasted the challah, they were once again filled with joy and hope. The Rabbi thought the congregation had grown because of his great sermons, and he was filled with his own rapture. After a year had passed, finances improved and the Rabbi quickly instructed his wife to stop her baking and to go and buy the challah from the best baker in town.

During that special time of the service, the Rabbi uncovered the perfectly baked loaves, proving he had overcome his poverty. But when he distributed to his congregation the pieces of challah from these perfectly braided, golden loaves, no one experienced the soulful joy they had when they had eaten the Rebbitsin's challah.

Soon people stopped coming. The Rabbi was confused and troubled. No one really knew what specifically had changed, but they did know that Shabbos with the Rabbi and Rebbitsin no longer brought a light into their lives. As the congregation diminished, so too did the finances, and the Rabbi could no longer afford the fancy breads. With anger and disdain he had to return to using the misshapen, sometimes scorched loaves that his wife baked. However, at the same time, he began to look inward at his own heart. He began to realize that it was not his words that brought joy to the people. As it always is, when we are in the greatest despair, truth begins to reveal itself.

After distributing the bread to his congregants, the Rabbi noticed the delight return to the faces of his followers as they ate the Rebbitsin's challah. There must be some magic, he thought to himself. My wife must be using a special ingredient.

Finally, one Friday morning he went to her and said that he wanted to watch and see how she made her challah. She was embarrassed, but she agreed to show him. He watched as she simply mixed flour, water, yeast, eggs, a little butter, sugar, and a pinch of salt on a wooden board. He watched as she put the dough in a bowl and covered it until the dough had risen. He saw nothing magical or special.

When the dough had risen, the Rebbitsin took out the dough and began to divide it into three lumps for braiding. She explained to her husband that while she rolls the first lump into a long strand, she meditates, thinking only of the Divine Name. She then takes a second lump of dough and said that she calls it her strand of contemplation, because as she rolls it, she contemplates the dough itself as a source of sustenance. "My thoughts just fly up to heaven of their own accord." Finally, the Rebbitsin took the last lump of dough and began rolling it smooth and long. She told the Rabbi that while she rolls this third piece of dough, she pours her prayers into it for their home, family, village, and all the suffering people of the world. She then took the three stands in her hands and showed him how she braided them together and put the loaf in the oven to bake. "You see," she said, "it's very simple."

That Friday evening the Rabbi seemed different. He spoke with humility, softness, and tenderness. His congregants even noticed that his hand trembled a bit when he lifted the Kiddish (wine) cup to pray. As he said the Ha-motzi, tears filled his eyes. He distributed the challah to everyone present and joined with them as they chewed their tiny bits of bread. This time his heart was filled with a joyful light and sweetness . . . a feeling he had never known before. With a full heart, the Rabbi wished the people a "Good Shabbos," inwardly grateful for the wisdom of his wife.

From that time on, people came far and wide to hear his wise teachings and heartfelt prayers . . . always filled with the joyful sweetness and light of the Rebbitsin's challah.

I think the philosophy behind Naomi's story is remarkably similar to that of Arun Gandhi's. Like the king who was given the mystery of life through a simple grain of wheat, so too was the Rabbi given the gift through the simple challah lovingly baked by his wife. Also, like the king, he could not see what was before him. He could only see a plain, misshapen loaf of bread. His golden box was his own ego—he walked around thinking *he* possessed the magic, but all the while he possessed *nothing*. We are not the keepers, we are the caretakers only. Like the words of the wise Indian sage who told the King that he has to plant the wheat, nurture it, take care of it, the Rebbitsin took her dough and kneaded it with love, prayer, compassion. And so it grew to feed the souls of those who ate of it.

What are the messages woven within the fabric of these stories? The answer lies within each of our hearts. For me, I think of my Bubbie and the way in which she took her time preparing the challah for us to enjoy. I wonder if she knew that it wasn't the ingredients themselves that made the challah so delicious as much as it was the spiritual ingredients of her love and prayers. Yes, it was a long time ago, but I still remember how my Bubbie kneaded the dough on our floured Formica table until it was smooth and soft and whole. Most of all, I remember how her delicate fingers would break off a piece of dough and gently hand it to me. Bubbie knew a lot about baking challah . . . I am still learning.

Steppingstone Nineteen

THE MEMORY BOTTLE

*"God must have realized that humans
need to be connected with the past,
so he gave us memories."*

—Mike Ruhland[11]

ftentimes we find ourselves sinking in the quicksand of negative or painful memories and need to have a meaningful way of
lifting ourselves out of that entrenchment. Being able to access positive memories is one way to help us achieve that endeavor.

I first read about a Memory Bottle in a moving story published in
Reader's Digest entitled "Message in a Starry Sky,"[12] written by Annette
Baslaw-Finger, a woman who courageously escaped the Nazi invasion
of her French homeland when she was just a child. The story was
given to me as a gift from one of the outreach workers with whom I
was fortunate to work within the Natural Healing Activities program
after Hurricane Iniki. Ms. Baslaw-Finger recounts how her father

called her over to him just before they had to make their way into a windowless cellar when the police were about to close in on the place where she and her family had been hiding.

Her "Papa" told ten-year-old Annette that they might have to stay in hiding for a long time. "We have to find ways to remember how special this world is," he said to her. She then describes how he "pretended to take an imaginary object off a shelf," and said, "Let's open a memory bottle. . . . We will put into it only the sights, smells, and moments that are most precious to us." He told her to remember the feeling of walking through the grass, the smells of different flowers, the color of the sky, and the feeling of the breeze. He concluded by telling her to put all of her memories into the bottle and put the cork in it. Little Annette did as her father suggested.

Whenever Annette felt despondent, her beloved Papa would tell her to "pull the cork and take out a memory." Sometimes she would take out a "patch of blue sky . . . the scent of a rose," which always made her feel better.

Since I read about the Memory Bottle, the story has become the seed from which a tangible experience has blossomed. I hope the same can happen for you. On the page provided, I invite you to create your own Memory Bottle and reconnect to the magic of positive memories in your own life, using these five simple steps as your guide:

1. Find some quiet, uninterrupted time and review in your mind a few positive memories in your life . . . experiences that are joyful to remember, such as a walk in the park with a special friend, the smell of your grandmother's home-baked bread, a holiday celebration, a random act of kindness someone showed you, a magical sunset, or a time when you achieved that I-can't-believe-I-did-it accomplishment.

2. After you have retrieved those special moments from your mental photo album, close your eyes and imagine a symbol that best represents each remembered experience. In a sense you are mentally creating a *logo* that represents your treasured experience. For example, whenever I think of my grandmother, I visualize a little grey and white bird.

3. With your eyes still closed, imagine a bottle that can hold these positive memories. Notice its shape, size, color.

4. When that image appears clearly in your mind, open your eyes and draw it on the following page.

5. Next, draw on your bottle the symbols from Step two that best represent your memories.

Annette Baslaw-Finger and her family arrived safely in Philadelphia on August 23, 1943. As an adult she earned her Ph.D. and became a foreign language professor. A proud grandmother of four, she has opened a Memory Bottle for each of her children and grandchildren. Although I have never met Dr. Baslaw-Finger—or her Papa—I am forever grateful to both of them for their story and their gift of memory and hope.

My Memory Bottle

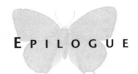

The Banana Kiss

"We come, we do, we go, and the doing
can be a rather grand voyage if you don't panic and
if you believe, as I believe, in magic and imagination
and wizards who live along quiet
country roads."

—Robert James Waller[1]

ave you ever met someone so magical that something about the encounter, no matter how brief, left you with a memory forever etched into the sacred spaces of your heart? Well, just such an encounter happened to me in May of 1991 during a lunch break from a conference I was teaching at Newington Children's Hospital in Connecticut. Dr. Jim Monahan, Director of Psychology, invited me to go on rounds with him to visit the children who were there for treatment. While walking through the hallways, we came upon an enchanting, copper-skinned girl of about five years of age who was sitting across from a nurse's station. She had a sunshine smile, large, round twinkling eyes the color of deep chocolate, and brown curly pigtails. Although she was strapped into a wheelchair and didn't seem to have the use of her lower body, she was able to talk and to use her upper body quite well. On her lunch tray was a half-eaten sandwich, two cookies, milk, and a banana. The nurse told me that she usually took a very long time to eat and indicated that perhaps I could encourage her to finish her lunch. I felt so captivated by the presence of this little pigtailed doll, that I filed the nurse's request away in the back of my mind. I squatted down to meet her at eye level. "Hello, my name is Joyce; what's your name?" I *thought* I heard her reply, "My name is Delores," so I responded by saying, "Delores, what a beautiful name." "NO," she snapped back at me, "My name is *not* Delores, my name is DEMORES!" "Ohhh," I replied. "Of course, Demores—that is even a better name just for you." She must have liked that response because little Demores twinked her eyes and flashed a bright smile back at me.

After talking with Demores a bit about what she liked to do and then about the delicious-looking lunch on her tray, she glanced toward an empty chair next to her, then she looked at me, then back at the empty chair. With a bit of pouting, a puffed-out lower lip, and a pleading tone in her voice, Demores said, "I surrre would like it if *someone* would keep me company . . . if *someone* would have lunch with me" . . . all the while glancing at the chair and then back at me. Demores repeated her suggestion again. I smiled as I inwardly thought, "Ah, the good-old Gestalt therapy 'empty-chair' technique and she never even took a formal class."

I glanced at Jim as if to ask if we had time to stay, but he signaled it was time for us to get back to the workshop. Not wanting to leave abruptly, I took the cookie she offered, and then I tried to employ a therapy approach that usually is effective in helping kids with separation. I asked if she had an imaginary friend or a favorite cartoon character who could keep her company. But you see, Demores was a lot smarter than me. Emphatically she shook her head and with a loud voice she said, "NO, I want a REAL somebody, not a make-believe somebody."

Jim then stepped in and explained to her that we had to go back to the auditorium, that I was there to teach about storytelling and that this was our special time to have a short visit with the children in the hospital, but that I couldn't stay. I also told Demores how much I wished I could sit and share lunch with her, but that I just couldn't stay. Inside I felt a secret wish that I could have fulfilled her request, but it truly was time for me to get going.

Before I left, I asked Demores if I could give her a good-bye kiss. "No," she said with a pouting tone. I then asked if I could perhaps throw her a kiss. With her pigtails swaying back and forth and her lips pursed together, she shook her head from side to side, indicating a definite "NO" once again. Of course, I realized that if she accepted the kiss it meant she would have to acknowledge the good-bye and she didn't want to do that . . . she wanted me to stay.

For some reason the uneaten banana on her tray drew my attention and sparked an idea. I told her that just in case she should want a kiss later, I would leave one for her in a special place. Demores looked at me with a lilt of curiosity as if to say, *"Now Joyce, how are you going to do that?"*

I then lifted the banana slowly, leaned all the way down, kissed the tray, and then gently replaced the banana over the kiss. Looking softly into her eyes I said, "You know, Demores, every once in a while everyone wants to have a kiss, so I'm gonna leave this kiss for you right here under the banana. Maybe sometime later, I don't know when, you may want it . . . and all you'll need to do is lift the banana and the kiss will be right there waiting for you. I waved good-bye, and as Jim and I began to walk away, I turned my head to glance back at the nurse's station where Demores was still sitting. Demores leaned toward the tray and looked curiously at the banana. Slowly she reached forward with her little hand, lifted the banana, and rested her cheek on the very spot where I had placed the kiss. Demores smiled a heartfelt smile, because of course, the kiss was there . . . just where I had left it.

That short time with Demores provided me with a moment of magic that will remain with me always. It showed me that during those times when we feel most unloved or alone, when we feel fear gripping our very souls, we need to remember to look for the reconnection to faith . . . to the magic of life . . . to our heartsongs . . . to our souls . . . because you see, the kiss *is* always there . . . we just have to take the time to look for it.

To All My Relations

References

Introduction

1. van der Post, Laurens (1980). *The Heart of the Hunter* (quote by D. H. Lawrence). New York: Harcourt Brace.

2. Estes, Clarrisa Pinkola (1992). *Women Who Run With the Wolves*. New York: Balantine.

3. Mills, Joyce C., & Crowley, Richard J. (1986). *Therapeutic Metaphors for Children and the Child Within.* Philadelphia, PA: Brunner/Mazel, a member of the Taylor & Francis Group.

Part I : Renewal From the Roots Up

1. Hawaiian Proverb

2. Dickinson, Emily (1890). "Hope." *Poems.*

3. van der Post, Laurens (1978). *Jung and the Story of Our Time.* New York: Penguin Books. (Originally published 1976 by the Hogarth Press, London)

4. Campbell, Joseph, with Moyers, Bill (1988). *The Power of Myth.* New York: Doubleday.

5. Hammerschlag, Carl A. (1993). *The Theft of the Spirit.* New York: Simon & Schuster.

6. Dossey, Larry (1993). *Healing Words: The Power of Prayer and the Practice of Medicine.* New York: HarperCollins Publishing.

7. Borysenko, Joan & Borysenko, Miroslav (1994). *The Power of the Mind to Heal.* Carson, CA: Hay House Inc.

8. van der Post, Laurens (1978). *Jung and the Story of Our Time.* New York: Penguin Books. (Originally published 1976 by the Hogarth Press, London)

9. Mills, Joyce C. & Crowley, Richard J. (1986). *Therapeutic Metaphors for Children and the Child Within.* Philadelphia, PA: Brunner/Mazel, a member of the Taylor & Francis Group.

10. Mills, Joyce C. (1993). *Gentle Willow: A Story for Children About Dying.* Washington, DC: Magination Press.

11. Mills, Joyce C. (1992). *Little Tree: A Story for Children with Serious Medical Problems.* Washington, DC: Magination Press.

Part II: Lessons Learned From the Natural World

1. Swain, James A. (1992). *Nature as Teacher and Healer.* New York: Villard Books.

2. Baylor, Byrd & Parnall, Peter (1978). *The Other Way to Listen.* New York: Charles Scribner's Sons.

3. Chopra, Deepak (1989). *Quantum Healing.* New York: Bantam Books.

4. Dossey, Larry (1993). *Healing Words: The Power of Prayer and the Practice of Medicine.* New York: HarperCollins Publishing.

5. Hammerschlag, Carl A. (1988). *Dancing Healers.* San Francisco: Harper & Row.

6. Hammerschlag, C. (1998). *The Go-Away Doll.* Phoenix: AZ: Turtle Island Press, Inc.

7. Northrup, Christiane (1994/95). *Women's Bodies, Women's Wisdom.* New York: Bantam Books.

8. Remen, Rachel Naomi (1996). *Kitchen Table Wisdom.* New York: Berkeley Publishing Group.

9. Siegel, Bernie S. (1986). *Love, Medicine, & Miracles.* New York: Harper & Row.

10. Siegel, Bernie S. (1998). *Prescriptions for Living.* New York: HarperCollins.

11. Weil, Andrew (1995). *Spontaneous Healing: How to Discover and Enhance your Body's Natural Ability to Maintain and Heal Itself.* New York: Knopf.

12. Muir, John, quoted in James. A. Swain (1992). *Nature as Teacher and Healer.* New York: Villard Books.

13. Chopra, Deepak (1993). *Creating Affluence: Wealth Consciousness in the Field of All Possibilities.* San Rafael, CA: New World Library.

14. Chopra, Deepak (1994). *The Seven Spiritual Laws of Success.* San Rafael, CA: Amber-Allen.

15. de Saint-Exupery, Antoine (1943). *The Little Prince.* New York: Harcourt, Brace & World.

16. Ornish, Dean (1990). *Dr. Ornish's Program for Reversing Coronary Artery Disease.* New York: Random House.

17. Angelou, Maya (1997). *Even the Stars Look Lonesome.* New York: Random House.

18. Dickinson, Emily (1890). "Cocoon Forth a Butterfly." *Poems.*

19. Walley, Paul (1988). *Butterfly & Moth.* New York: Eyewitness Books—Alfred A. Knopf.

20. Paulus, Trina (1972). *Hope for the Flowers.* New York: Paulist Press.

21. Thoreau, Henry David—Journal, August 23, 1853. Quoted in James. A. Swain (1992). *Nature as Teacher and Healer.* New York: Villard Books.

22. Giono, Jean (1985). *The Man Who Planted Trees.* Chelsea, VT: Chelsea Green Publishing Company.

23. Angelou, Maya (1997). *Even the Stars Look Lonesome.* New York: Random House.

24. McNally, David (1990). *Even Eagles Need a Push.* New York: Delacorte Press.

Part III: Restoring the Breath of Life

1. van der Post, Laurens (1992). *About Blady: A Pattern Out of Time.* New York: William Morrow.

2. Ovid, *Metamorphoses,* XV, 252-255; as cited in Joseph Campbell (1976). *The Hero with a Thousand Faces,* Bollingen XVII, 2nd edition, revised. Princeton, NJ: Princeton University Press.

3. Momaday, N. Scott (1992). *In the Presence of the Sun: Stories and Poems, 1961-1991.* New York: St. Martin's Press.

4. Feng, Gia-Fu and English, Jane (1972). *Tao Te Ching; Lao-tzu: A New Translation.* New York: Vintage Books (a division of Random House).

5. Proverbs 4:23.

6. Lee, Pali J. & Willis, Koko (1990). *Tales of the Night Rainbow.* Night Rainbow Publishing, P.O. Box 10706, Honolulu, HI.

7. Nestel, Fran (1996). *Ka Ipu Kukui* (The Bowl of Light)—A picture-songbook: Honolulu HI: Night Rainbow Publishing.

8. van der Post, Laurens (1972). Epigraph in *A Story Like the Wind.* New York: Harcourt Brace Javanovich, Publishers.

9. Kushner, Lawrence (1994). *Honey From the Rock.* Woodstock, VT: Jewish Lights Publishing.

10. Zukow, Bud and Sayles, Nancy (1996). *Baby: An Owner's Manual. A Beloved Pediatrician Answers Your First 365 Phone Calls.* New York: Kensington Books.

11. Estes, Clarrisa Pinkola (1992). *Women Who Run With the Wolves.* New York: Balantine.

12. Hanh Nhat, Thich (1990). *Present Moment, Wonderful Moment.* Berkeley, CA: Parallex Press.

13. Hillel. *Pirke Avot I:14.*

Part IV: Rituals and Ceremonies for Remembering What Deserves to Be Cherished

1. Burne-Jones, E. C., to Wilde, Oscar (1880).

2. Tucker III, Gershon A. (1993). Personal communication to CharlesEtta Sutton.

3. Gibran, Kahlil (1976). *The Prophet.* New York: Alfred A. Knopf.

4. *Little Miracles.* (1996-1998). Quote by Thomas Carlyle. Edmonds, WA: Compendium Press.

5. Hammerschlag, Carl A. & Silverman, Howard D. (1997). *Healing Ceremonies.* New York: A Perigree Book—The Berkley Publishing Group.

6. Sen, Shoshitsu XV (1979/76). *Tea Life, Tea Mind.* New York: John Weatherhill, Inc.

7. Doe, Mimi and Waller, Garland. (1995). *Drawing Angels Near.* New York: Pocket Books (a division of Simon & Schuster, Inc.).

8. Mills, Joyce C. (1989). *Stories of the Dreamwalkers* (Limited Edition). Distributed by author. Kekaha, HI.

8a. Mills, Joyce C. (1998). Personal quote.

9. Hanh Nhat, Thich (1976/87). *The Miracle of Mindfulness.*(Translated by Mobi Ho). Boston: Beacon Press.

10. Doe, Mimi & Waller, Garland (1995). *Drawing Angels Near.* New York: Pocket Books (a division of Simon & Schuster, Inc.).

11. Remen, Rachel Naomi (1996). *Kitchen Table Wisdom.* New York: Berkeley Publishing Group.

Part V: Giveaway . . . Sharing the Vision

1. Carter, Forrest (1976). *Education of Little Tree.* Albuquerque, NM: University of New Mexico Press.

2. *Little Miracles.* (1996-1998). Quote by Anne Frank. Edmonds, WA: Compendium Press.

3. Hammerschlag, Carl A. (1988). *Dancing Healers.* San Francisco: Harper & Row.

4. *Little Miracles.* (1996-1998). Quote by Mother Teresa. Edmonds, WA: Compendium Press.

5. Looking Horse, Arvol (1996). "Letter for World Peace and Prayer Day."

6. van der Post, Laurens. (1987). *Walk with a White Bushman.* New York: William Morrow.

7. Gandhi, Arun (1996). "Non-Violence or Nonexistence: Options for the 21st Century." A keynote presentation for National Speakers Association.

8. Siegel, Bernie S. (1998). *Prescriptions for Living.* New York: HarperCollins.

9. Gibran, Kahlil (1976). *The Prophet.* New York: Alfred A. Knopf.

10. Steinberg, Naomi (1995).*The Dybbuk and Other Stories for Reading Aloud.* Naomi Steinberg Publisher, P.O. Box 274, Carlotta, CA 95528.

11. *Little Miracles.* (1996-1998). Quote by Mike Ruhland. Edmonds, WA: Compendium Press.

12. Baslaw-Finger, Annette (1993). "Message in a Starry Sky," in *Reader's Digest—November, 1993.* Pleasantville, NY: The Reader's Digest Association.

Epilogue

1. Waller, Robert J. (1994). *Old Songs in a New Cafe*. New York: Warner Books.

Recommended Readings

Canfield, Jack & Hansen, Mark V. (1993-99). *Chicken Soup for the Soul*. Deerfield Beach, FL: Health Comunications, Inc.

Crowley, Richard J. & Mills, Joyce C. (1989). *Cartoon Magic: How to Help Children Discover TheirRainbows Within*. Washington, DC: Magination Press.

Dalai Lama (1991). *Worlds in Harmony: Dialogues on Compassionate Action*. Berkeley, CA: Parallax Press.

Horn, Sam (1996). *Tongue Fu*. New York: St. Martin's Press.

Horn, Sam (1998). *Concrete Confidence*. New York: St. Martin's Press.

Little Miracles. Cards with inspirational quotes. Compendium Inc., P.O. Box 912, Woodinville, WA 98072. 1-800-IDEAS.

Loomis Todd, Mabel & Higginson, T. W. (Edited original editions). (1992). *Collected Poems of Emily Dickinson*. New York: Gramercy Books.

Mills, Joyce C. & Crowley, Richard J. (1988). *Sammy the Elephant and Mr. Camel*. Washington, DC: Magination Press.

Napier, Nancy J. (1997). *Sacred Practices for Conscious Living*. New York: W. W. Norton & Company.

Napier, Nancy J. (1993). *Getting Through the Day*. New York: W. W. Norton & Company.

Osbon, Diane K. (Ed.) (1991). *Reflections on the Art of Living: A Joseph Campbell Companion*. New York: Harper Perennial.

Pottiez, Jean-Marc (Ed.) (1994). *Feather Fall* (Quote by Laurens van der Post). New York: William Morrow & Company.

Resources

The Turtle Island Project is a nonprofit organization dedicated to a vision of health and healing. For more information regarding our Healing Journey Retreats please contact:

>The Turtle Island Project
>5624 W. Edgemont Avenue
>Phoenix, AZ 85035
>Phone: (520) 318-7210 (West Coast Office)
>(908) 753-9489 (East Coast Office)
>E-mail: buttrfly@gte.net

The mission of the M. K. Gandhi Institute for Nonviolence is to teach and apply the principles of nonviolence as a positive force to PREVENT violence and resolve personal and public conflict.

>M. K. Gandhi Institute for Nonviolence
>Christian Brothers University
>650 E. Parkway South
>Memphis, TN 38104
>Arun Gandhi, Founder Director
>(901) 452-2824.
>E-mail: gandhi@odin.cbu.edu

The Milton H. Erickson Foundation, Inc., provides educational programs designed for professionals in the health sciences. The purpose of the Foundation is to further the worldwide understanding and practice of medical and clinical hypnosis and hypnotherapy by promoting in every ethical way the contributions made to the field by the late Milton H. Erickson, M.D.

>The Milton H. Erickson Foundation, Inc.
>3606 North 24th Street
>Phoenix, AZ 85016-6500

Executive Director: Linda Carr McThrall
(602) 956-6196
E-mail: office@erickson-foundation.org

The vision and endeavor are for all people from all cultures and beliefs to come together and pray for global healing.

Chief Arvol Looking Horse
World Peace and Prayer Day
P.O. Box 421
Spearfish, SD 57783
www.worldpeace.com/1999

The Landmine Survivors Network is a nonprofit organization created by American land-mine survivors to help the hundreds of thousands of civilian land-mine victims, and to prevent new ones from joining their ranks.

Landmine Survivors Network
700 Thirteenth St. NW, #950
Washington, DC 20005
Tel: (202) 661-3537
Fax: (202) 661-3529
E-mail: LSN@landminesurvivors.org

The mission of the Sophia Center is to provide a safe and affirming environment for women and men to explore the journey of feminine consciousness through spirituality and creativity, thus transforming work, family, community, and the sacred dimension of their lives.

Sophia Center
P.O. Box 128
Marylhurst, OR 97036
Sister Katherine Knoll, Director
(503) 636-5151

The International Institute of Applied Consciousness provides workshops and seminars that "facilitate the world in living and playing at its highest level of consciousness."

International Institute of Applied Consciousness
5025 N. Central Avenue, #240
Phoenix, AZ 85012
(602) 252-3249
E-mail: a298@amug.org

Play Therapy International makes training available for child psychotherapists and play therapists. It is a philosophy of this organization that every effort must be made to bring programs to developing countries and to offer programs to citizens of developing countries at a cost that would not in any way be prohibitive.

Play Therapy International
I IE - 900 Greenbank Road, Ste. 527
Nepean (Ottawa), Ontario,
K2J 4P6, Canada
Mark A. Barnes, Ph.D., Director
(613) 634-3125
E-mail: celtic@full-moon.com

You Are Invited

I am of the belief that we can never have enough stories. They are the gifts and legacies we share with all. If you have an inspirational short story of your own that you feel matches the spirit of this book, and would like to share it with others, I invite you to send it to me for possible inclusion in a future book entitled *Butterfly Magic Stories*. If selected, you retain all rights to your story for you to use in any other publications or personal projects. Please send the story, a short biographical paragraph, and your address, phone/fax number/E-mail address to:

Joyce C. Mills, Ph.D.
Imaginal Press
P.O. Box 1109
Kekaha, Kaua'i, HI 96752

Speaking and Training Information

For information regarding speaking engagements, consulting work, and training programs, please contact me at the address, phone/ fax number, or E-mail address mentioned below. All presentations are designed to meet the personal needs of your group. Follow-up consultations and small group trainings are available upon request.

Joyce C. Mills, Ph.D.
Breakthrough Seminars
P.O. Box 1030
Kekaha, Kaua'i, HI 96752
Phone/FAX: (808) 337-9551
E-mail: buttrfly@gte.net

Thank you for your interest and support, and remember that the *Magic* is there when we just take the time to look for it.

With Aloha,
Joyce C. Mills

A Gift from the Author to You

Dear Reader,

  I would like to offer you a free colorful bookmark that has five principles for enhancing *Self Appreciation* printed on it. To receive this special gift, send your name and mailing address, along with a self-addressed stamped #10 (11 inches long) envelope, and a bookmark will be sent directly to you. For every name and stamped, self-addressed envelope, I will be delighted to send a complimentary *Self Appreciation* bookmark.

  Please send all requests to:

Imaginal Press
P.O. Box 1109
Kekaha, Kaua'i, HI, 96752